Mechanical Support of the Failing Heart and Lungs

Mechanical Support of the Failing Heart and Lungs

EDITED BY

David Bregman, M.D.

Assistant Professor of Surgery
Columbia University
College of Physicians and Surgeons
New York, New York

APPLETON-CENTURY-CROFTS/New York

ACC

Library of Congress Cataloging in Publication Data

Main entry under title:

Mechanical support of the failing heart and lungs.

Papers presented at conference, June 5, 1976.
Includes index.
1. Blood--Circulation, Artificial--Congresses.
2. Oxygenators, Membrane--Congresses. I. Bregman, David. (DNLM: 1. Heart, Mechanical--Congresses. 2. Extracorporeal circulation--Congresses. 3. Heart surgery--Congresses. 4. Assisted circulation--Congresses.
WG168 M486 1976)
RD598.M45 617'.412 77-4165

77 78 79 80 81 / 10 9 8 7 6 5 4 3 2 1

Prentice-Hall International, Inc., London
Prentice-Hall of Australia, Pty. Ltd., Sydney
Prentice-Hall of India Private Limited, New Delhi
Prentice-Hall of Japan, Inc., Tokyo
Prentice-Hall of Southeast Asia (Pte.) Ltd., Singapore
Whitehall Books Ltd., Wellington, New Zealand

PRINTED IN THE UNITED STATES OF AMERICA

Contributors

HENRIK H. BENDIXEN, M.D.
Professor and Chairman
Department of Anesthesiology
Columbia University
College of Physicians and Surgeons
New York, New York

FREDERICK O. BOWMAN, JR., M.D.
Associate Professor of Clinical Surgery
Columbia University
College of Physicians and Surgeons
New York, New York

DAVID BREGMAN, M.D.
Assistant Professor of Surgery
Columbia University
College of Physicians and Surgeons
New York, New York

RICHARD A. DE ASLA, B.A.
Bio Engineer
Division of Cardiothoracic Surgery
Mount Sinai School of Medicine
of the City University of New York
New York, New York

RICHARD N. EDIE, M.D.
Assistant Professor of Surgery
Columbia University
College of Physicians and Surgeons
New York, New York

ADAM FISCHER, M.D.
Resident
Division of Cardiothoracic Surgery
Mount Sinai School of Medicine
of the City University of New York
New York, New York

HILLARD L. FITZKEE, B.S.
Bio Engineer
Division of Cardiothoracic Surgery
Mount Sinai School of Medicine
of the City University of New York
New York, New York

PIERRE M. GALLETTI, M.D.
Professor of Medical Science
Brown University
Division of Biological and Medical Sciences
Providence, Rhode Island

VINCENTE GRANA, M.D.
Instructor of Surgery
Mount Sinai School of Medicine
of the City University of New York
New York, New York

SUSAN M. HAUBERT, R.N.
Chief Clinical Perfusionist
Columbia University
College of Physicians and Surgeons
New York, New York

J. DONALD HILL, M.D.
Senior Research Member
Heart Research Institute
Institute of Medical Science
Pacific Medical Center
San Francisco, California

ROY A. JURADO, M.D.
Assistant Professor of Surgery
Mount Sinai School of Medicine
of the City University of New York
New York, New York

ROBERT M. KOFFSKY, B.S., M.S.
Bio Engineer
Division of Cardiothoracic Surgery
Mount Sinai School of Medicine
of the City University of New York
New York, New York

FOUAD A. LAJAM, M.D.
Assistant Professor of Surgery
Mount Sinai School of Medicine
of the City University of New York
New York, New York

ROBERT S. LITWAK, M.D.
Professor of Surgery and Chief
Division of Cardiothoracic Surgery
Mount Sinai School of Medicine
of the City University of New York
New York, New York

SALVADOR B. LUKBAN, M.D.
Assistant Professor of Surgery
Mount Sinai School of Medicine
of the City University of New York
New York, New York

JAMES R. MALM, M.D.
Professor of Clinical Surgery
Chief, Chest Surgical Service
Columbia University
College of Physicians and Surgeons
New York, New York

JOHN C. NORMAN, M.D.
Clinical Professor of Cardiothoracic Surgery
The University of Texas Medical School at San Antonio
San Antonio, Texas;
Director of Cardiovascular Surgical Research Laboratory
Texas Heart Institute
Houston, Texas

ARCADIO F. ORTIZ, M.D.
Instructor of Surgery
Mount Sinai School of Medicine
of the City University of New York
New York, New York

GEORGE PAPPAS, M.D.
Associate Professor of Surgery
University of Colorado Medical Center
Denver, Colorado;
Chief of Cardiovascular Surgery
Denver Veterans Administration Hospital
Denver, Colorado

EDUARDO N. PARODI, M.D.
Senior Research Associate
Columbia University
College of Physicians and Surgeons
New York, New York

E. CONVERSE PEIRCE, II, M.D.
Henry Kaufman Professor of Hyperbaric Surgery
Mount Sinai School of Medicine
of the City University of New York
New York, New York

KEITH REEMTSMA, M.D.
Professor and Chairman
Department of Surgery
Columbia University
College of Physicians and Surgeons
New York, New York

JAMES J. SHERMAN, A. B.
Research Fellow
Division of Cardiothoracic Surgery
Mount Sinai School of Medicine
of the City University of New York
New York, New York

GEORGE SILVAY, M.D.
Assistant Professor
Department of Anesthesiology
Mount Sinai School of Medicine
of the City University of New York
New York, New York

HENRY M. SPOTNITZ, M.D.
Assistant Professor of Surgery
Columbia University
College of Physicians and Surgeons
New York, New York

PETER P. STEELE, M.D.
Professor of Medicine
University of Colorado
Medical School
Denver, Colorado;
Chief of Cardiology
Veterans Administration Hospital
Denver, Colorado

ROBERT SZARNICKI, M.D.
Chief Resident in Cardiothoracic Surgery
Columbia University
College of Physicians and Surgeons
New York, New York

WARREN M. ZAPOL
Assistant Professor of Anesthesiology
Harvard Medical School
Boston, Massachusetts

Contents

Foreword

The advent of cardiopulmonary bypass in 1953 and further refinements established the specialty of cardiovascular surgery, allowing repair of acquired and complex congenital cardiac defects. The support system as now constituted is imperfect, limited in time of life support, and variable in the distribution of blood flow during circulatory support to myocardium, major organs, and muscle mass. The regional distribution of myocardial blood flow in particular has been shown to be variable. A means of providing cardiac and circulatory support for prolonged periods of time without the need for anticoagulation or invasive techniques would be ideal. The quest for such a system to meet pre- and postoperative clinical problems has produced a number of inventive and ingenious approaches. Systems of supporting circulation and the failing heart represent a new frontier in a developing specialty. The more recent developments in the area have brought together engineers, scientists, and physicians in a collaborative effort to approach the problem of the prolonged and physiologic support of the circulation.

The direction has led into two paths: (1) the development of an artificial lung for oxygenation suitable for meeting total oxygen consumption following acute respiratory insufficiency; (2) use of support devices directed toward reducing cardiac work, particularly left ventricular work, and improving myocardial perfusion during surgery and in the recovery period. Total prolonged circulatory support is the ultimate goal in the quest for the ideal mechanical system to preserve life during a transition or holding period.

The present book is a publication of papers presented at a conference on this subject June 5th, 1976. It represents the latest information and developments presented by authorities in this field, the new frontier in cardiac surgery.

James R. Malm, M.D.

Mechanical Support of the Failing Heart and Lungs

CHAPTER 1

Pulsatile Cardiopulmonary Bypass

George Pappas
Peter P. Steele

Pulsatile blood flow for isolated organ and total cardiopulmonary bypass perfusion has been reported to be superior to that found with nonpulsatile flow.[1] Current pulsatile pumps have not been used to any extent because of their unreliability, hazards, and complexity.[2] The use of intra-aortic balloon pumping (IABP) for the treatment of cardiogenic shock from a variety of causes has gained recent popularity. Berger and Saini[3] demonstrated in dogs that IABP during cardiopulmonary bypass (CPB) converts a nonpulsatile CPB (NPF) to that of pulsatile flow (PF). This technique was also explored independently of their findings in the animal laboratory and has been used clinically.[4,5,6]

In addition, we investigated the concept of infant CPB and coronary artery pulsatile perfusion. The infant intra-aortic balloon (4.5 cc) was tested in animals, as well as developing a bolster pulsatile pump for pulsatile infant and coronary artery perfusion.

METHODS AND MATERIALS

Since May 8, 1973, we have employed the technique of IABP during CPB in adult patients which demonstrated a physiologic pulse contour. Details concerning balloon insertion and activation have been previously described.[1,4,7] During our initial experience, we inserted the balloon in a retrograde fashion from the femoral artery. The disadvantages with this approach include an additional arteriotomy (with its inherent complications) and difficulties of insertion, which indicate that it may be a hazardous procedure. We elected to use an alternate antegrade approach by inserting the balloon in the distal ascending aorta and positioning the balloon just beyond the left subclavian artery.[7] This approach has been used in nearly all of our more recent patients because of its simplicity and expedience. It is important to explore the descending thoracic aorta to rule out disease and assure proper balloon position. We have been surprised on occasion to discover an unexpected thoracic aneurysm or atheromatous disease precluding this approach. It is also *essential* that bilateral carotid artery compression be applied by the anesthesiologist to make certain that the balloon does not traverse these vessels. We have had this happen on two occasions, and proper reinsertion was necessary. Balloon activation can be achieved by the electrocardiogram (ECG) or external pacing depending on the particular needs.

Arterial pressure tracings and doppler flow (Fig. 1) recordings

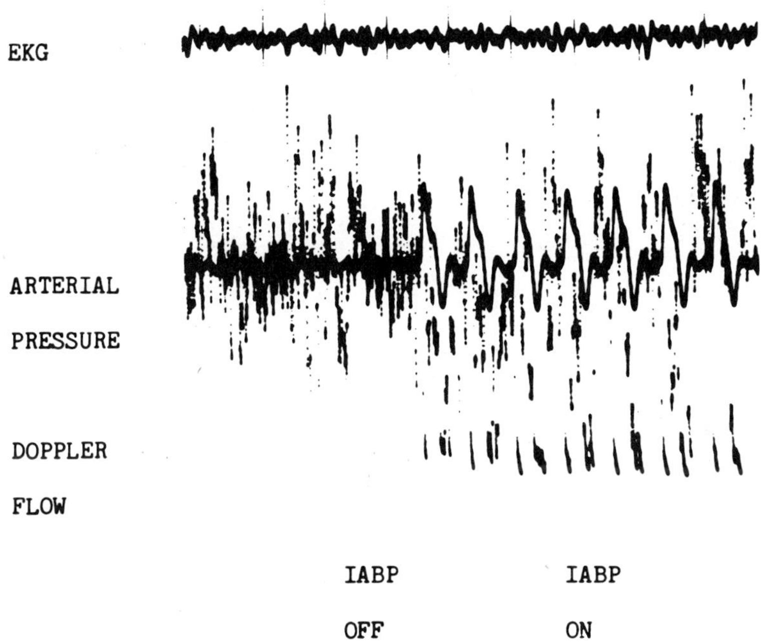

FIG. 1. Comparison of arterial pressure contour and Doppler flow during nonpulsatile cardiopulmonary bypass (left) and pulsatile flow using IABP (right).

demonstrate physiologic pulsatile CPB. In addition, palpation of the aorta and saphenous vein bypass grafts during IABP produce pulsations that can be seen and felt. Frequently, pulsatile bleeding is seen with open coronary arteries. A trisegment AVCO* intra-aortic balloon was used because of its sequential inflation and dispersion of the pulse wave in both directions as confirmed by similar pressure recordings obtained at the femoral and radial artery sites. In adult patients, pulsatile flow occurs with the balloon inflated to from 15 to 20 cc. Larger volumes for the most part do not augment pressure recordings and may (although it has not been documented) produce obstruction at the balloon site.

The infant balloon (4.5 cc) has been investigated in the laboratory in dogs. The balloon characteristics included are a displacement of 4.5 cc (volume), a length of 114.3 mm, a diameter of 8.55 mm when fully inflated, and mounting on a No. 7 French catheter. It does produce a pulsatile flow as measured by carotid

**Hoffman-LaRoche, Inc., Cranbury, N.J.*

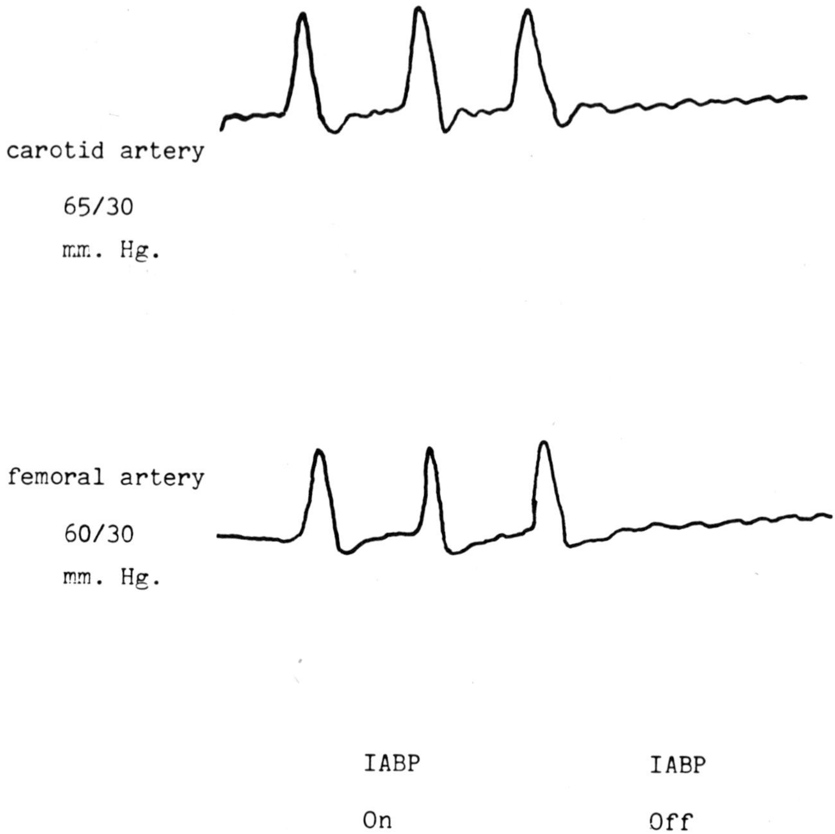

FIG. 2. Arterial pressure recordings demonstrating pulsatile flow using the 4.5 cc infant balloon (left) and the nonpulsatile flow (right) in a large-sized dog.

and femoral arterial pressure tracings (Fig. 2). However, at times, especially in small dogs (5 to 8 kg), obstruction to flow at the balloon site occurs when using arterial perfusion via the ascending aorta (Fig. 3).

A second and different method of producing pulsatile flow was investigated in the animal laboratory using a bolster pulsatile pump. The system consists of attaching in series, a Waters* pulsatile pump (model PC101) attached to the arterial line between the roller pump and the arterial cannula (Fig. 4). The arterial tubing is placed within the compressing heads of the Waters pump

**Waters Corp., Rochester, Minn.*

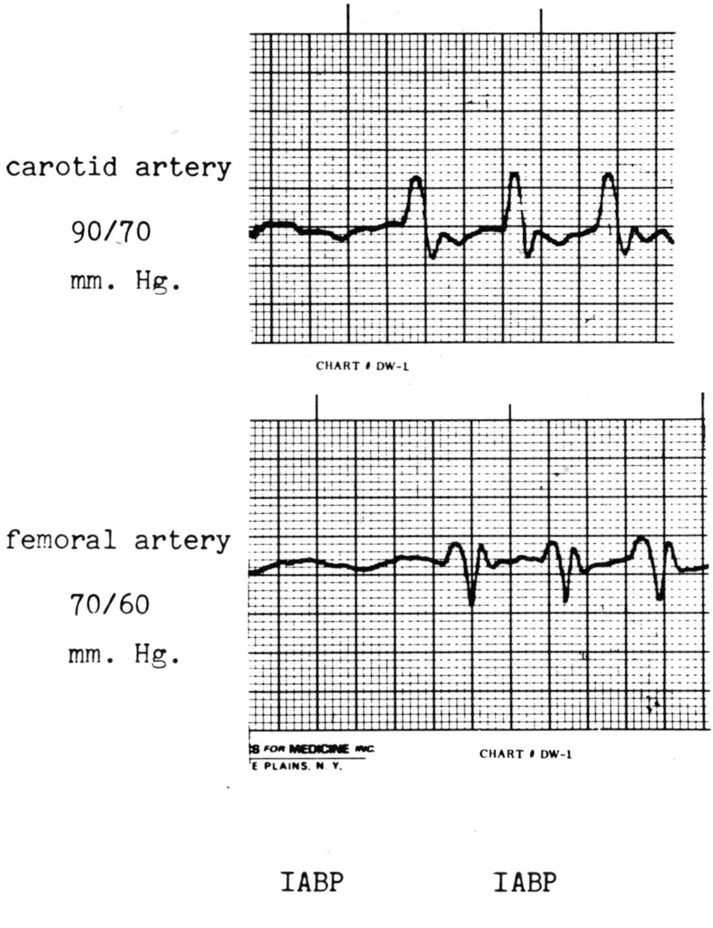

FIG. 3. Arterial pressure recordings with a 4.5 cc infant balloon during cardiopulmonary bypass in a smaller dog. Note the lack of pulsatile flow beyond the balloon (probably due to obstruction) as demonstrated by the femoral artery tracing.

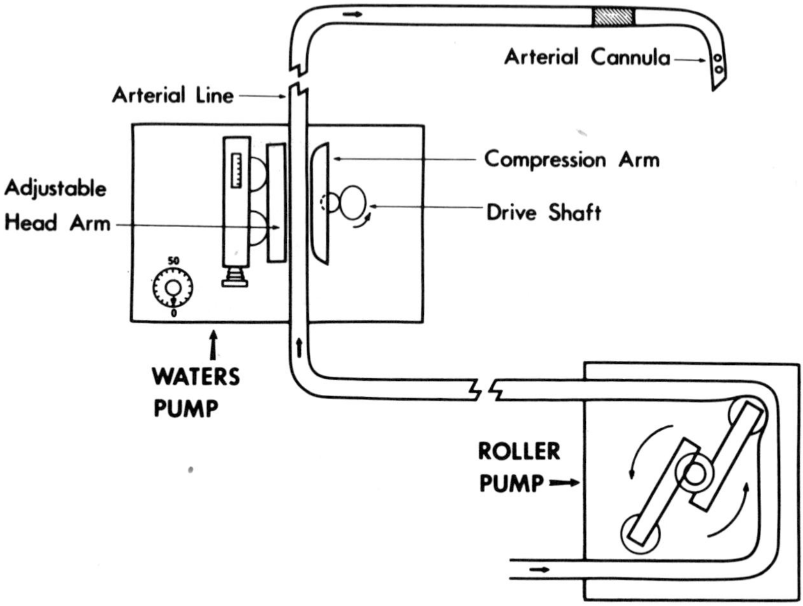

FIG. 4. Schematic diagram demonstrating the valveless bolster pulsatile pump. Pulsatile flow can be produced by simple compression of the arterial line.

without the need of valves. Simple compression of the tubing resulted in a forward displacement of blood toward the arterial cannula and retrograde wave, which stops at the roller pump head. For coronary perfusion in dogs, 1/4-inch internal diameter I.D. Tygon* tubing was used. Coronary artery pressure tracings demonstrated pulsatile flow (Fig. 5). The same system using 3/8-inch I.D. Tygon tubing was tested for pulsatile CPB in dogs. The principle was clinically applied in October, 1973, in five infant open cardiac procedures demonstrating a pulse contour (Fig. 6). The bolster pulsatile pump demonstrated pulsatile flow at flows between 30 to 1500 ml/ minute. Cardiopulmonary bypass flows beyond 1500 ml/minute pulsations did not occur, probably due to the rapid transit of blood through the tubing.

Details in metabolic and myocardial function studies have been previously reported in man using IABP and CPB.[1,5,6] Comparisons were made in a similar group of adult patients not receiving pulsatile flow. Moderate hypothermia (30 C) was used in

**Norton Co., Akron, Ohio.*

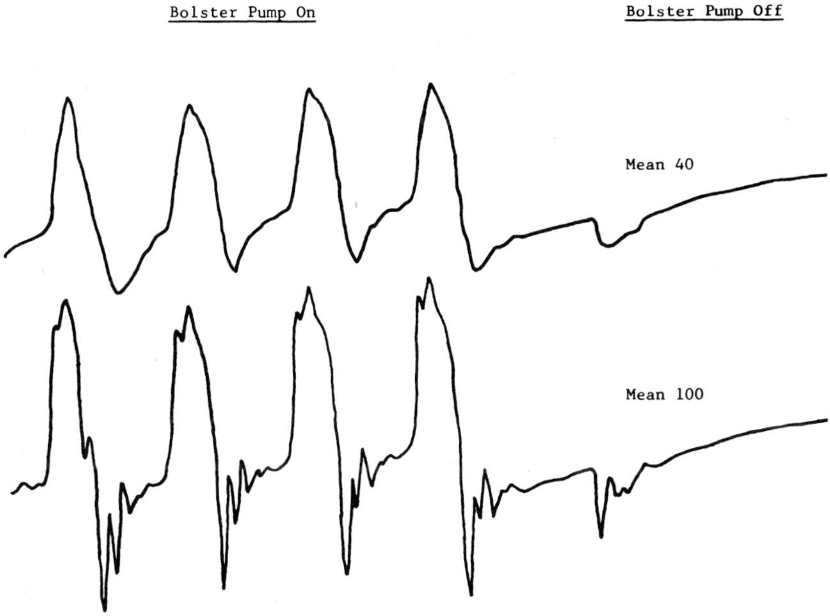

FIG. 5. Arterial pressure recordings of a dog's left anterior descending coronary artery and arterial perfusion line using coronary perfusion. Note the pulsatile flow (PF) produced by the bolster pulsatile pump (left) and nonpulsatile flow (right). A 110 mm Hg systolic gradient was present across the coronary artery cannula during PF. Left coronary flow = 80 cc per minute. Top, LAD (mm Hg) 100/60; bottom, coronary perfusion arterial line (mm Hg) 210/80.

all patients. With coronary artery bypass (CAB) procedures, the aorta was not clamped and coronary bleeding was controlled by local compression, tourniquets, or balloon catheters. Ventricular fibrillation was used in all coronary artery bypass patients who were studied. All aortic anastomoses were done prior to CPB. Studies consisted of coronary sinus myocardial lactate changes, production, extraction, and "excess," and O_2 extraction and coronary sinus arterio-venous (AV) O_2 difference during CPB. Immediate postoperative left ventricle (LV) function was determined by a radionuclide technique of measuring LV ejection fraction (LVEF) in a comparable group of 20 NPF and 20 PF coronary bypass patients. This technique employs the use of ^{113m}Indium given into a central vein and recorded by a precordial collimated scintillation probe. The details of the procedure and results have been previously described.[8,9] In addition, serum glutamic-oxaloacetic transaminase (SGOT), total lactic dehydrogenase (LDH), and plasma hemoglobin were also studied postoperatively.

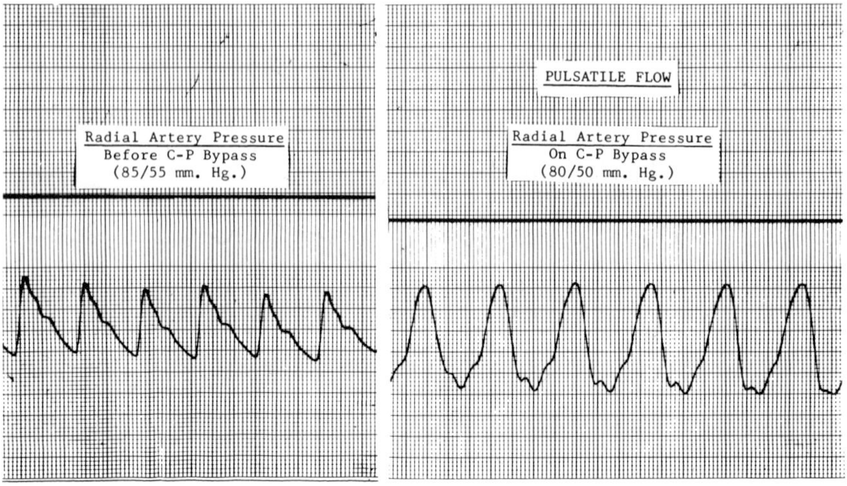

FIG. 6. Arterial pressure recordings using the bolster pulsatile pump during cardiopulmonary bypass in a pediatric patient during a Mustard repair. Note the patient's own arterial pressure (left) and the pressure contour (right) produced by the bolster pulsatile pump.

CLINICAL MATERIAL

IABP and CPB

This form of pulsatile flow was used in 182 patients having bypass procedures or valve replacement(s). In 107 patients, the balloon was inserted into the distal ascending aorta. There were 55 low-risk patients consisting of single CAB (6, nearly all with internal mammary artery bypasses), double CAB (17), triple CAB (29), and mitral valve replacement or repair (3). There were 127 "high-risk" patients receiving pulsatile flow, 76 had left ventricular dysfunction (LVEF less than 0.40). The conditions treated are listed in Table 1.

Bolster Pulsatile Pump

There were five infants who had pulsatile CPB using a bolster pump in tandem with the arterial line (Fig. 4). The congenital lesions treated are listed on Table 2.

TABLE 1. Pulsatile CPB in High Risk Patients

AMI, CGS, VSD, or MVR*	3
Left main CAD†	24
Preinfarction angina	31
CAB and LV‡ dysfunction	36
LV aneurysmectomy	5
Prolonged CPB§–Valve and CAB (4–6)	16
Reop CAB	8
AVR‖ (renal failure)	1
MVR	3
Total	127

**AMI: acute myocardial infarction; CGS: cardiogenic shock; VSD: ventricular septal defect; MVR: mitral valve replacement.*
†CAD: coronary artery disease.
‡CAB: coronary artery bypass; LV: left ventricle.
§CPB: cardiopulmonary bypass.
‖AVR: aortic valve replacement.

TABLE 2. Pulsatile CPB (Bolster Pump) in Infancy

	CASE 1	CASE 2	CASE 3	CASE 4	CASE 5
Lesion	VSD	DTGA,IS*	DTGA,IS	VSD,PDA	VSD,PA band
Repair	Patch	Mustard	Mustard	Patch PDA	Deband PA; patch
Age (mo)	12	18	11	12	24
Wt (kg)	5.3	8.0	8.5	6.1	11
CPB duration (min)	60	102	100	56	75
CPB flow (cc/min)	600	800	1000	700	1200
CPB pressure	65/25	80/50	70/45	95/65	70/48
Plasma Hb (mg%)†	52	192‡	76	93	87
Outcome	Survived	Survived	Survived	Died§	Survived

**DTGA,IS (dextrotransposition of the great arteries, intact ventricular system).*
†Post CPB.
‡Considerable intracardiac suction.
§Stable hemodynamics, cardiorespiratory arrest 24 hours postoperatively while changing endotracheal tube.

RESULTS

IABP and CPB

There were eight operative deaths in 182 patients receiving pulsatile CPB (4.4 percent). The cause of deaths included arrhythmias (two patients), acute myocardial infarction (AMI) following CPB (two patients), massive preoperative AMI (one patient), balloon perforation of a normal common iliac artery with shock, AMI and CAB (one patient), sepsis and renal failure starting two weeks postoperative (one patient), and massive pulmonary embolism and cardiac failure (one patient). There were four late deaths (2.3 percent): two from arrhythmias and two noncardiac deaths. The remaining patients have been followed from 6 to 37 months (mean, 17 months).

Bolster Pulsatile Pump

In five infants, the bolster pulsatile pump was used during CPB. The clinical conditions and data collected are shown in Table 2. These patients were operated on in 1973, and as with other infant perfusions, hemolysis was not infrequent, which cleared within a matter of hours. A similar degree of hemolysis was noted in our pulsatile patients. In each patient, we were able to produce a pulse contour (Fig. 6). However, there was one operative death. This patient was hemodynamically stable with a clear and adequate urine output. Problems developed with the endotracheal tube 24 hours postoperatively, and cardiorespiratory arrest occurred while changing the tube. Hemodynamics deteriorated despite supportive measures.

Metabolic and Functional Studies (adult patients)

Pulsatile flow patients (CAB, aneurysmectomy, mitral valve procedures) were compared with nonpulsatile patients. These studies have been previously described.[1,5,6,9] There were significantly greater differences in coronary sinus lactate changes, production, extraction, and "excess lactate" found in NPF versus PF patients. There were no significant differences in myocardial O_2 studies (extraction and AV O_2 differences) noted, though the results appeared more stable in the PF group. Total LDH and SGOT were lower in PF patients versus NPF. The degree of postoperative hemolysis was similar in both groups. The LVEF was significantly elevated during the immediate postoperative period (days 1 to 12) in the PF patients having CAB procedures, whereas it was depressed in the NPF group. In two small subgroups of patients with perioperative AMI and left main coronary disease, LVEF rose in the PF patients and fell in the NPF. A larger number of patients need studying in these subgroups before definitive conclusions can be reached about the technique of perfusion.

Analysis of the ECGs in for new Q waves (perioperative infarctions) were made in 235 patients having CAB procedures.[9] The incidence of perioperative infarctions was 7.3 percent in 8 of 109 patients with PF versus 11.1 percent in 14 of 126 NPF patients (P less than 0.05). We tended to use PF in patients requiring more saphenous vein grafts and who had poorer left ventricular function, and in a significant number of patients with high-risk preinfarction angina. In 55 patients presenting with congestive heart failure and angina pectoris, we thought that pulsatile flow may improve late myocardial performance.[6] Detailed studies of cardiac performance, progression of coronary disease, graft patency, etc, need assessing to substantiate or disprove this finding.

DISCUSSION

Standard CPB with nonpulsatile flow has been the acceptable method for open cardiac procedures. Pulsatile CPB has not been used to a great extent in man because previously developed pulsatile pumps were not generally accepted for a variety of reasons (complexity, hemolysis, unreliability, etc). The advantages of PF versus NPF for isolated organ perfusion and total body perfusion have been documented by many investigators.[1] Unfortunately, the ideal pulsatile pump has not been developed. We have explored pulsatile perfusion in two ways, namely, for use of IABP during CPB and for the development of a valveless bolster pulsatile pump.

Our previous studies of using IABP with CPB in adult patients have demonstrated its superiority to that of standard perfusion.[1,5,6,9] In using this technique for PF, the benefits derived should be balanced against possible disadvantages, such as an added surgical procedure with its potential complications. It is our feeling that there are advantages in pulsatile perfusion, especially in patients requiring prolonged CPB, or with depression of myocardial or other vital organ function. There was only 1 complication out of 182 patients (0.6 percent). The balloon was inserted via the femoral artery which resulted in perforation of a *normal* common iliac artery. This could have been easily avoided were it inserted gently. In some patients, it was difficult or impossible to insert the balloon from the groin. Under these circumstances, we have recently been inserting the balloon into the distal ascending aorta (antegrade approach) in 107 patients without a complication. However, it is important that caution be applied during insertion: bilateral carotid pressure should be applied so that the balloon does not extend up these vessels. Palpitation of the aortic arch and descending aorta is also important to rule out arterial disease.

We found that IABP served several purposes. The antegrade approach is a rapid method of insertion in those patients with deteriorating hemodynamics. We have adopted the technique of inserting the proximal saphenous vein grafts on the aorta first while the patient is cannulated and not on bypass. Inserting the IABP beforehand probably results in benefits of diastolic augmentation and decreased left ventricular work while performing the aortic anastomoses. Balloon pumping is continued during CPB triggered by an external pacemaker or the patient's ECG. In more recent patients, we have allowed the heart to beat with synchronous augmentation during the coronary anastomoses while on CPB. Theoretically, it would appear that diastolic augmentation during moderate hypothermia (30 C) in an empty beating heart should provide optimal protection to the myocardium. However, hard data are not available to support this hypothesis.

The IABP can also be used to wean the patient from cardiopulmonary bypass without the need of supportive drugs with their potential hazards. During the pulsatile CPB, we have found that the mean arterial pressure in the majority of patients does not increase with the passage of time. In NPF patients, increased arterial pressure secondary to an increased peripheral vascular resistance was frequently observed. Because of the lowered peripheral vascular resistance with PF, we think that some patients may be supersensitive to protamine infusion. In a couple of patients, profound shock was associated with protamine infusion, which necessitated reinstitution of CPB. Having observed this phenomenon, we have used IABP during and for at least 15 minutes following protamine infusion. The hypotensive effect was easily counteracted. When hemodynamics became stable the balloon was removed.

We have utilized this simple form of pulsatile flow in patients with depressed myocardial function, high-risk preinfarction angina, multiple valve replacement, cardiogenic shock, left ventricular aneurysm resection, etc. For obvious reasons, the only condition in which this system is not applicable is during isolated aortic valve replacement. However, PF may provide protection to other malfunctioning vital organs (brain, kidney, liver, etc). Previous studies from this institution suggest that PF is better than NPF with regard to myocardial metabolism and function, perhaps because of less hepatocellular injury (postoperative SGOT levels), better overall tissue perfusion (total LDH), lower incidence of perioperative myocardial infarction, and possible improvement in late myocardial function. Postoperative renal failure (necessitating diuretics, etc) has been rare in our experience. This is in contrast to a recent study by Abel et al,[10] who found that 27 percent of their patients had mild to severe renal failure, which correlated with the duration of CPB, aortic crossclamp time, and the total duration of operation.

We tended to use PF in potentially high-risk patients. The use of IABP before, during, and following CPB may have some influence on the overall outcome. Excluding those patients with preoperative or pre–CPB cardiogenic shock (six patients), four patients (2.3 percent) required postoperative support. Three of the four had severe left ventricular dysfunction preoperatively. In the remaining 173 patients, postoperative low cardiac output (ie, myocardial injury) was not observed, therefore, inotropic drugs and diuretics were not needed. The operative mortality rate of 4.4 percent and the late mortality rate of 2.3 percent are not unreasonable when considering all the cardiac lesions treated.

In a pilot study using the infant intra-aortic balloon (4.5 cc) in dogs, pulsatile flow during CPB was demonstrated. In some dogs, however, especially those with a small aorta, pulsatile flow distal to the balloon did not occur. It is our impression that the lack of pulsatile flow beyond the balloon resulted from obstruction at the balloon site or the inability of the pump console to properly deflate the balloon. Both the femoral and ascending aortic approaches were used for balloon insertion. From our experimental studies, pulsatile flow using the current infant balloon is not indicated in patients less than 5 to 8 kg because of the obstruction phenomenon and the potential injury to small femoral arteries. It is noteworthy that in some dogs postmortem studies demonstrated that the balloon when inflated was of similar diameter to the descending aorta. This may be a factor responsible for the obstructive process. A small balloon with a small catheter size and a more effective balloon control system may prove beneficial for future clinical use in infants. The 4.5 cc balloon may prove effective for larger subjects (20 kg). It has not been tested in larger animals. Coarctation of the aorta and interrupted aortic arch are obvious contraindications for the use of this technique in infants or children.

The second system of valveless pulsatile flow using a Waters pulsatile pump with the roller pump in tandem, does produce a pulse contour in both coronary perfusion and CPB in small subjects. Pulsatile flow was proven experimentally and was used in five infants requiring open cardiac procedures. Postoperative hemolysis in our patients did not differ substantially from that seen with standard CPB. There were no complications associated with this procedure. Further experimental and clinical use is necessary to evaluate the system in detail. The attractive feature of this technique is its valveless nature, and if mechanical or electrical failures were to occur, the pump could be turned off and standard perfusion resumed. The system employed is nonsynchronous, but we are currently constructing a synchronous pump which may provide the advantages of counterpulsation.

SUMMARY

Our studies indicate that pulsatile CPB using IABP appears better than standard CPB. Pulsatile CPB in adults improves myocardial metabolism and performance, reduces the incidence of myocardial injury, may improve the flow to other vital organs, and may show long-term improvement of myocardial function in comparison to nonpulsatile flow. Only one complication occurred in 182 patients (incidence of 0.6 percent) using the IABP. There have been no complications using the antegrade ascending aortic approach in 107 patients. The use of the infant intra-aortic balloon (4.5 cc) needs further experimental evaluation and modification before it can be applied to neonates or infants. Its application and precautions have been outlined.

A second method of external pulsatile perfusion (bolster pulsatile pump) is presented. This technique works only at low flow states (ie, 30 to 1500 cc/minute), beyond which the system is ineffective. The pump system is valveless, and if failures were to occur, the pump can easily be discontinued and standard perfusion resumed. This technique may be used for both coronary perfusion as well as pediatric perfusion. The bolster pulsatile pump was used in five open pediatric cardiac procedures without a complication. Further evaluation of this technique appears warranted.

REFERENCES

1. Pappas G, Steele P, Paton BC: A simple method of producing pulsatile flow during clinical cardiopulmonary bypass using intraaortic balloon pumping. In Norman JC (ed): Coronary Artery Medicine and Surgery. New York, Appleton, 1975, p 478
2. Trinkle JK, Helton NE, Wood RE, Bryant LR: Metabolic comparison of a new pulsatile pump and a roller pump for cardiopulmonary bypass. J Thorac Cardiovasc Surg 58:562, 1969
3. Berger RL, Saini VK: Conversion of nonpulsatile cardiopulmonary bypass to pulsatile flow by intraaortic balloon pumping during myocardial revascularization for cardiogenic shock (abstract). Circulation 46 (Supp. II):130, 1972
4. Pappas G: A simple method of producing pulsatile flow during clinical cardiopulmonary bypass. Ann Thorac Surg 17:405, 1974
5. Pappas G, Winter SD, Kopriva CJ, Steele PP: Improvements of myocardial and other vital organ function and metabolism with a simple method of pulsatile flow (IABP) during clinical cardiopulmonary bypass. Surg 77:34, 1975
6. Pappas G: Pulsatile flow during open heart surgery. In Davila JC (ed): Second Henry Ford Hospital International Symposium on Cardiac Surgery. New York, Appleton, 1977
7. Pappas G: Intrathoracic intraaortic balloon insertion for pulsatile cardiopulmonary bypass. Arch Surg 109:842, 1974
8. Steele PP, Van Dyke D, Trow RS, et al: Simple and safe bedside method for serial measurement of left ventricular ejection fraction, cardiac output and pulmonary blood volume. B Heart J 36:122, 1974
9. Maddoux G, Pappas G, Jenkins M, et al: Comparison of pulsatile and nonpulsatile flow during cardiopulmonry bypass on left ventricular ejection fraction early after aorto-coronary surgery. Am J Cardiol 37: 1000, 1976
10. Abel RM, Buckley MJ, Austen WG, et al: Etiology, incidence and prognosis of renal failure following cardiac operations. J Thorac Cardiovasc Surg 71:323, 1976

CHAPTER 2

Unidirectional Intra-Aortic Balloon Pumping and Counterpulsation During Open Heart Surgery

David Bregman
Eduardo N. Parodi
Susan M. Haubert
Robert Szarnicki
Richard N. Edie
Henry M. Spotnitz
Frederick O. Bowman, Jr.
Keith Reemtsma
James R. Malm

Supported in part by National Institutes of Health Research Grant No. 12738.

In recent years, the development of modern direct techniques for revascularization surgery has resulted in a multitude of critically ill patients undergoing open heart surgery. To deal with the increasing numbers of patients who require both urgent open heart surgery and who present with many complicated patterns of disease, a spectrum of cardiac assist measures ranging from simple

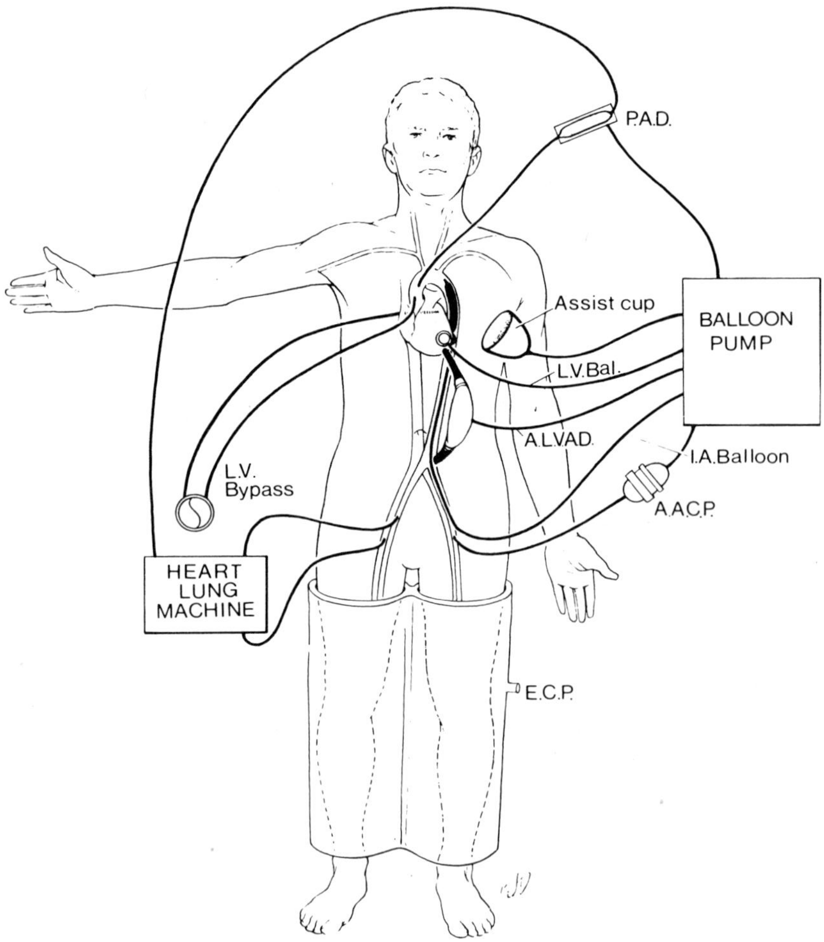

FIG. 1. Schematic of current clinical temporary mechanical cardiac assist techniques. LV, left ventricular; PAD, pulsatile assist device; IA balloon, intra-aortic balloon; ALVAD, abdominal left ventricular assist device; AACP, arterioarterial counterpulsation; ECP, external counterpulsation.

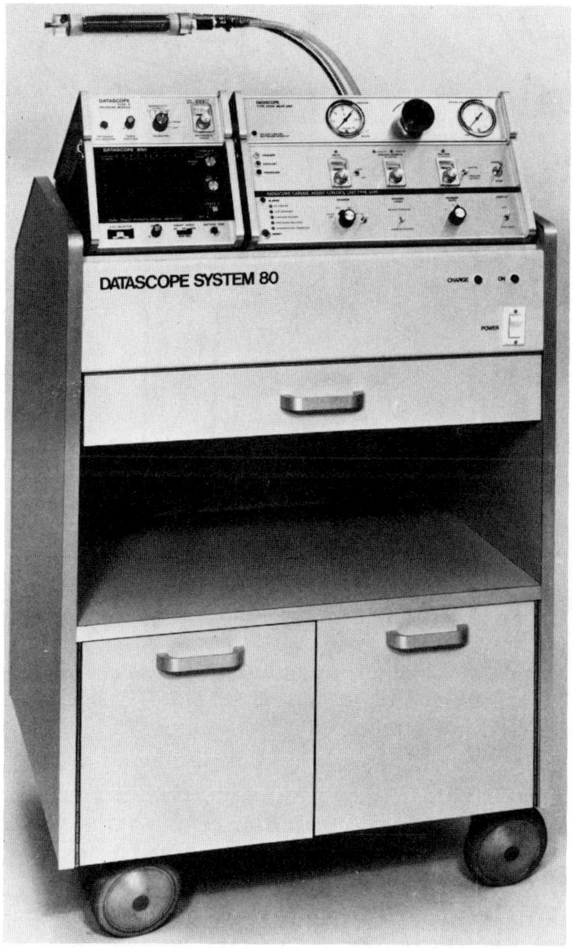

FIG. 2. Datascope System 80, a failsafe, mobile, cardiac assist console for balloon pumping.

pharmacologic interventions to the employment of several invasive mechanical cardiac assist techniques have been developed (Fig. 1). Those temporary mechanical cardiac assist devices which employed the principle of counterpulsation and balloon pumping have met with the most consistent clinical success. In particular, the intra-aortic balloon pump has now emerged as the temporary mechanical cardiac assist technique of choice for the management of refractory left ventricular power failure.[1,2]

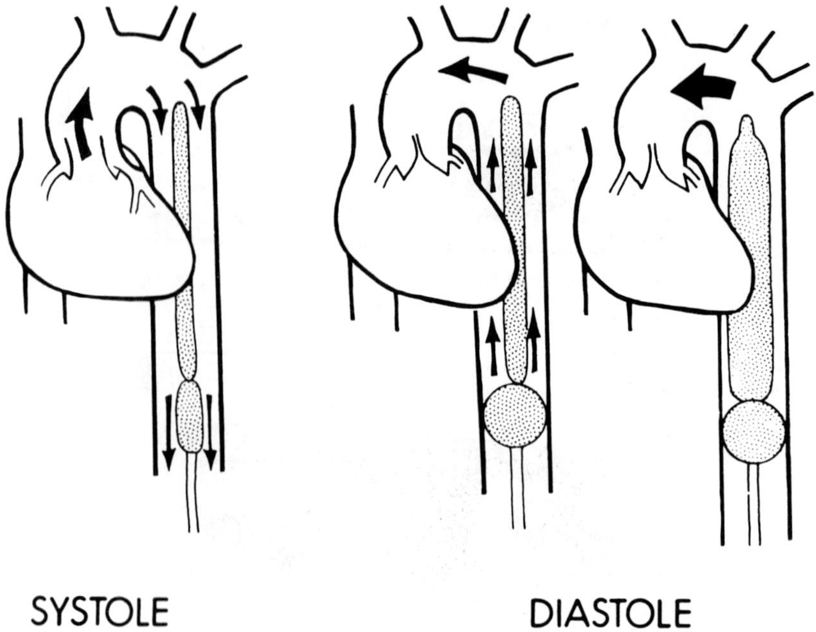

FIG. 3. Schematic illustrating the mechanism of action of a unidirectional dual-chambered intra-aortic balloon.

Prior to the institution and use of counterpulsation techniques in open heart surgery, left ventricular power failure and refractory ventricular arrhythmias had been associated with a mortality in excess of 90 percent after open heart surgery.[3,4] This chapter will detail our clinical results in patients with such complications after open heart surgery at the Columbia Presbyterian Medical Center in New York City. In addition, a new application of counterpulsation with pulsatile bypass as a routine adjunct to open heart surgery will be described. Finally, our experience with other types of potentially useful balloons will be discussed.

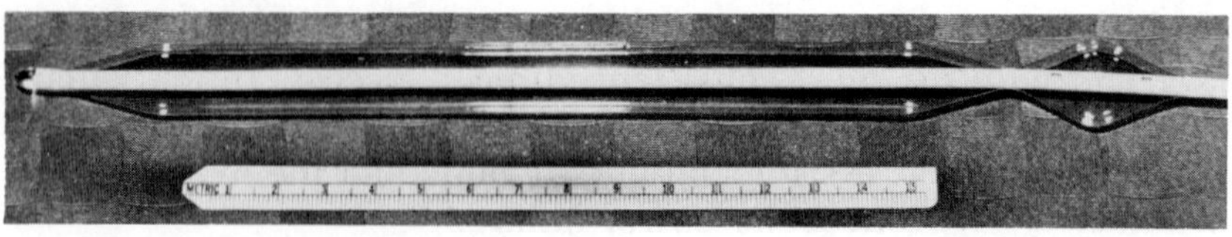

FIG. 4. Clinical unidirectional dual-chambered intra-aortic balloon (30 cc).

PATIENT SELECTION

In the 50-month period from Feb. 1, 1972, through April 30, 1976, 981 adult patients had corrective open heart surgery at the Columbia Presbyterian Medical Center. Of these patients, 63 underwent unidirectional intra-aortic balloon pumping (IABP) in conjunction with open heart surgery during that period. The average age of these patients was 55 years (range, 15 to 68 years) and the sex distribution was 43 men and 20 women.

The patients undergoing intraaortic balloon pumping were categorized under three separate groups:

Group A: The 17 patients in this category had either crescendo angina refractory to medical therapy or were in a low cardiac output state or in cardiogenic shock prior to cardiac catherization, and all of the latter patients were New York Heart Association class IV. Angiography would have been extremely hazardous in these individuals; therefore, IABP was instituted prior to their studies. IABP was continued throughout the catherization and into the postoperative period.

Group B: This group consisted of 30 patients in whom cardiopulmonary bypass could not be discontinued after cardiovascular surgery despite maximum pharmacologic support. All patients in this category had evidence of inadequate systemic perfusion, a high left ventricular filling pressure, the need for excessive inotropic drugs, or refractory ventricular tachyarrhythmias.

Group C: The 16 patients in this category were all assisted in the open heart recovery room within the first 24 hours following open heart surgery. All of these patients exhibited the progressive clinical picture of a low cardiac output syndrome consisting of arterial hypotension, a high left atrial or central venous pressure, and a markedly decreased urinary output, in spite of a requirement for high-dose inotropic support.

MATERIALS AND TECHNIQUES

The Datascope system 80* (Fig. 2), a mobile failsafe battery-operated cardiac assist console, was used to drive the

**Datascope Corp., Paramus, N.J.*

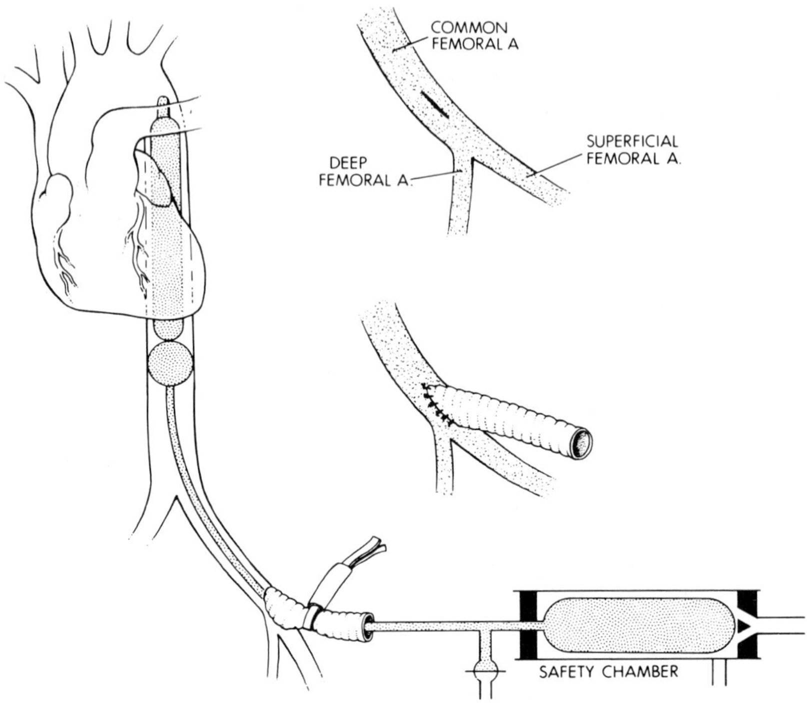

FIG. 5. Schematic representation of clinical dual-chambered IABP.

intra-aortic balloon.[5] Pumping was effected from the R wave of the electrocardiogram, which triggered deflation of the intra-aortic balloon followed by inflation during diastole; thus, balloon inflation never coincided with ventricular systole. A unidirectional dual-chambered intra-aortic balloon (30 or 35 cc) was used exclusively in these studies (Figs. 3, 4).[6,7] The balloon was a spherical distal chamber which inflates early in diastole and occludes the aorta. This is sequentially followed by the inflation of a narrower cylindrical proximal balloon, in the same diastolic interval, which pumps intra-aortic blood entirely toward the aortic root. Both chambers are completely deflated by an active vacuum just prior to ventricular ejection.

The balloon was passed through the common femoral artery of the extremity with the stronger pulse and was positioned just distal to the left subclavian artery (Figs. 5, 6). A Dacron side-arm graft was sutured to the common femoral artery, and the graft and balloon catheter were snared so that the distal extremity would be

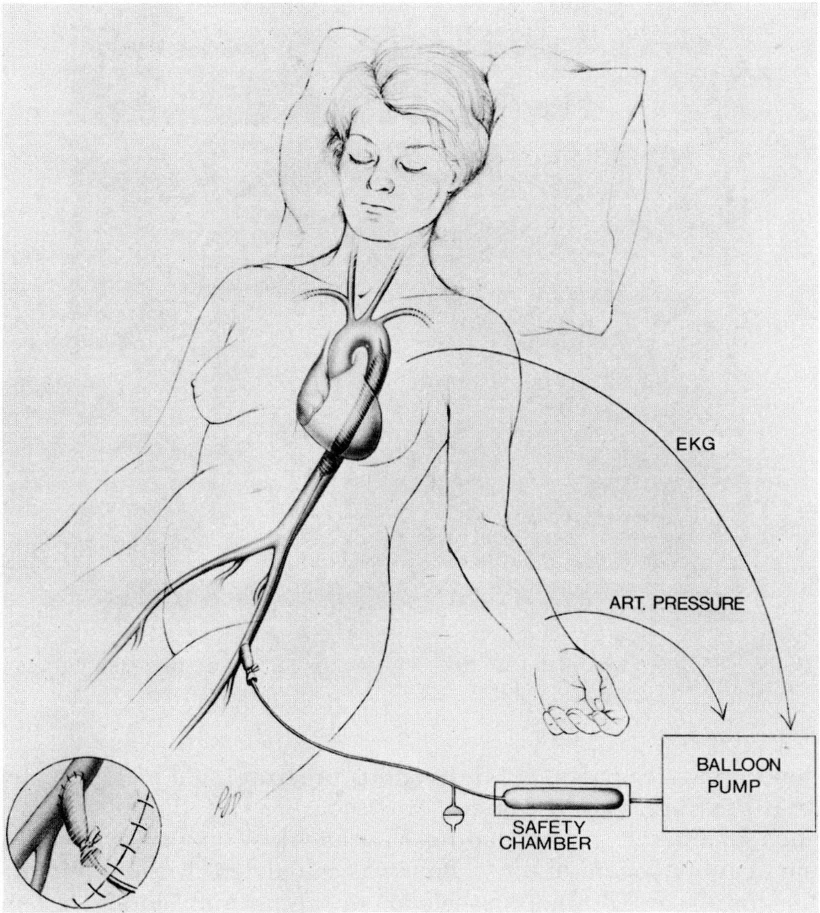

FIG. 6. Clinical schematic of balloon pumping after insertion.

perfused during the period of cardiac assistance.[7] In the group A patients, intravenous aqueous heparin was administered in a dose of 5000 to 7500 units every four to six hours. In the intra- and postoperative patients, aspirin, given rectally (600 mg every four hours), was utilized as the sole "anticoagulant" in these patients. When the balloon was removed, a Fogarty catheter was passed proximally and distally, and then a 1 cm stump of the graft was oversewn and left as a patch graft. Additional details of patient management have been described previously.[8]

Hemodynamic parameters were monitored, including arterial

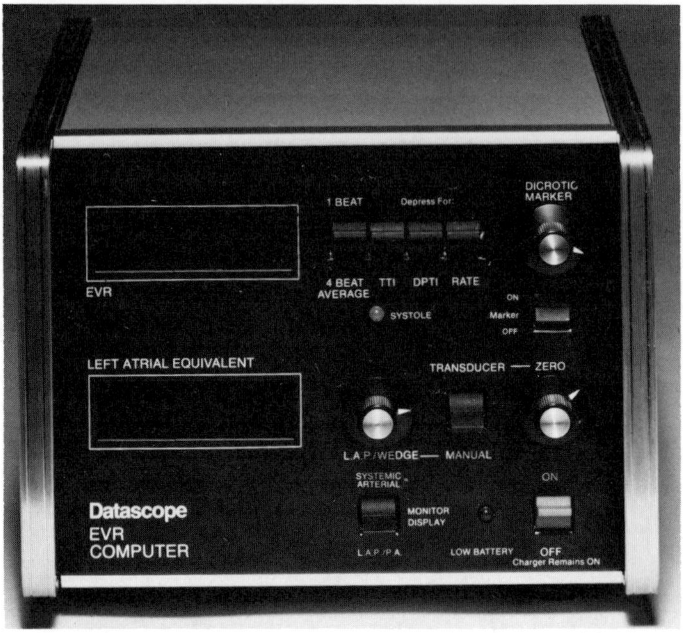

FIG. 7. EVR (endocardial viability ratio) computer for on-line monitoring of DPTI/TTI ratio.

blood pressure, pulse, central venous pressure, and wedge or left atrial pressure. Cardiac output was measured by thermodilution[9] when practical,* as were coronary graft blood flows.† An indication of subendocardial blood flow was calculated by the method of Buckberg[10] and Philips[11] by means of the ratio diastolic pressure time index tension/tension time index (DPTI/TTI). An analogue computer (Fig. 7)‡ was used to measure the area under the systolic (TTI) and diastolic (DPTI) radial artery pressure curve, to subtract the left atrial (or wedge) pressure from the DPTI, and to calculate the ratio DPTI/TTI, with a digital display of the result as the endocardial viability ratio (EVR). This computation has been shown to represent a reliable indication of the adequacy of subendocardial blood flow. An EVR of less than .8 implies subendocardial ischemia.[10,11]

**Edwards Laboratories, Inc., Santa Ana, Calif.*
†Carolina Medical Electronics, Inc., Winston-Salem, N.C.
‡Manufactured by the Datascope Corp., Paramus, N.J.

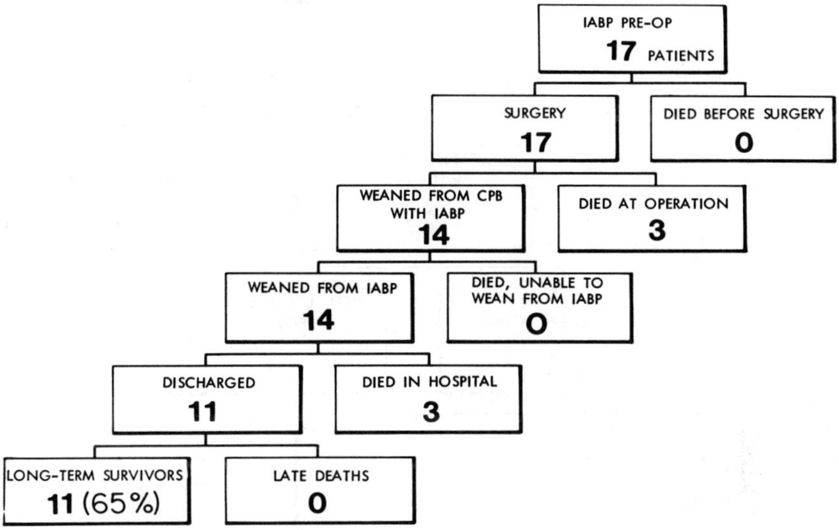

FIG. 8. Preoperative unidirectional intra-aortic balloon pumping (IABP), Columbia Presbyterian Medical Center, 1972–76: Group A. CPB, cardiopulmonary bypass.

RESULTS

Group A: The 17 patients in this group were assisted an average of 13 hours prior to open heart surgery (Fig. 8). These patients all underwent uneventful cardiac catheterization with balloon support and were assisted an average of 69 hours postoperatively. With the onset of balloon pumping, the pulmonary artery wedge pressures fell an average of 15 mm Hg. Urinary outputs increased an average of 49 cc in the first hour of support, and the mean arterial pressure increased 23 mm Hg. There was a marked decrease in the need for concurrent inotropic support. Of these patients, 11 were long-term survivors (65 percent). The disease entities encountered in these patients included refractory congestive heart failure with ventricular aneurysms, patients with crescendo angina refractory to medical therapy, patients with acute ventricular septal defects or acute mitral regurgitation after an acute myocardial infarction, and patients in the early stages of cardiogenic shock. There were no late deaths in this group.

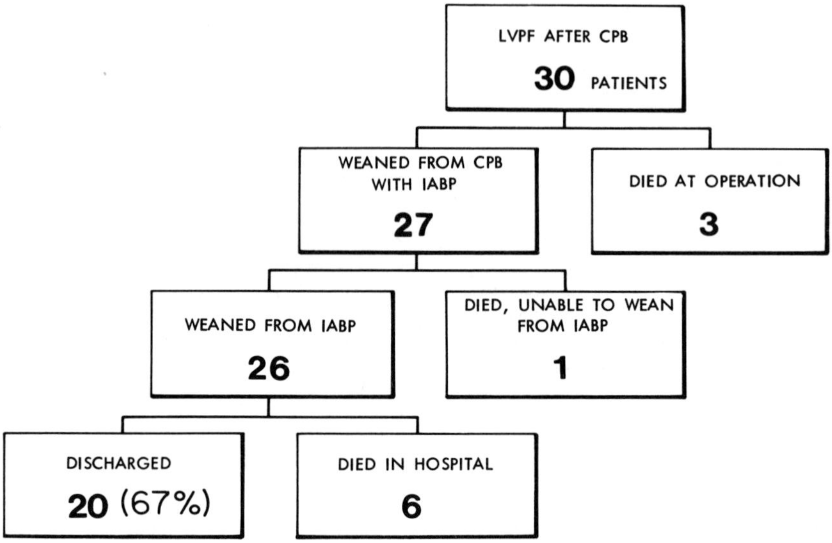

FIG. 9. Intraoperative unidirectional intra-aortic balloon pumping (IABP) Columbia Presbyterian Medical Center, 1972–76: Group B. LVPF, left ventricular power failure; CPB, cardiopulmonary bypass.

Group B: The 30 patients in this category were assisted for an average of 41 hours after open heart surgery (Fig. 9). Twelve patients incurred an acute intraoperative myocardial infarction, and three of these patients died. All three had diffuse subendocardial infarction of the left ventricle at autopsy.

IABP effected an average rise in mean arterial pressure of 41 mm Hg. Left atrial pressure fell an average of 16.5 mm Hg in those patients who were weaned from cardiopulmonary bypass.

Eight of the patients had ventricular tachyarrhythmias after bypass which were resistant to high doses of antiarrhythmic drugs. The cessation of arrhythmias in this group was striking, and an example is shown in Figure 10.

Twenty-seven of the thirty patients in this group were successfully weaned from cardiopulmonary bypass, and twenty (67 percent) were discharged from the hospital.

The intraoperative responses of coronary graft blood flow to unidirectional IABP, which were measured in 12 of the group B patients, showed a uniform increase in coronary blood flow in all patients when balloon assistance was instituted.[1,2] After the patient was weaned from cardiopul-

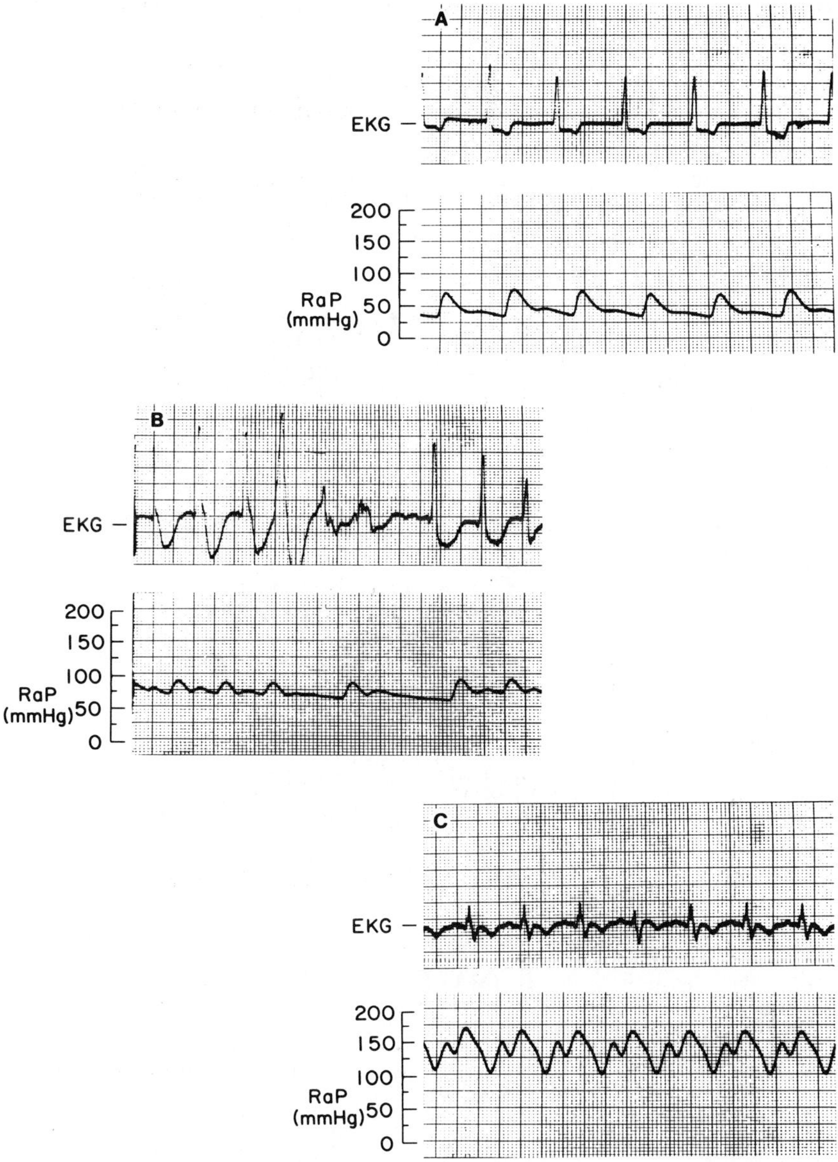

FIG. 10. Serial data on a patient who underwent aortic valve replacement for congenital aortic stenosis and incurred an acute intraoperative inferior wall myocardial infarction. A. Tracing taken immediately before institution of cardiopulmonary bypass. B. Tracing shows inability to wean patient from cardiopulmonary bypass after aortic valve replacement. Note ventricular tachyarrhythmias. C. Tracing taken 1 minute after the start of unidirectional intra-aortic balloon pumping and the cessation of cardiopulmonary bypass. Note the absence of arrhythmias. EKG, lead II of the electrocardiogram; RaP, radial artery blood pressure; tracing speed, 25 mm/sec.

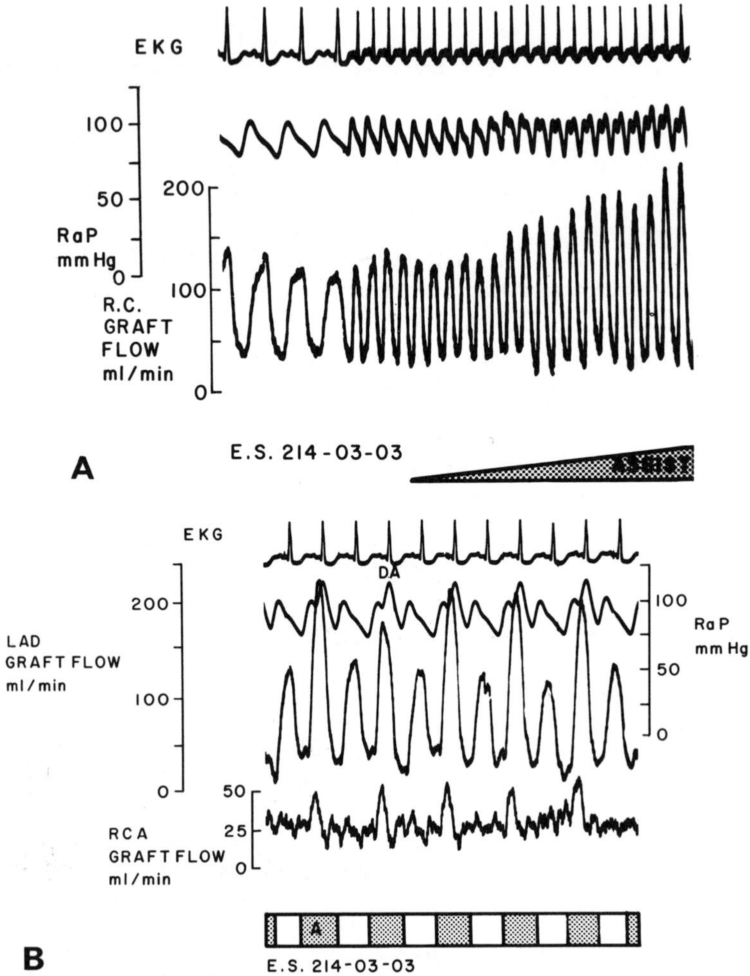

FIG. 11 A. Dual-chambered IABP in a patient assisted after aortocoronary bypass graft surgery. Flows were measured with a square-wave electromagnetic flowmeter. Note gradual continuous increase in RC graft flow as the balloon is gradually inflated to its maximum volume. B. With patient assisted every other beat, note the 100 percent increase in LAD and RCA graft flows during diastole. Tracing speed, 25 mm per second. A, assist (IABP) periods; DA, diastolic augmentation; LAD, left anterior descending coronary artery; RaP, radial artery pressure; RC, right coronary artery.

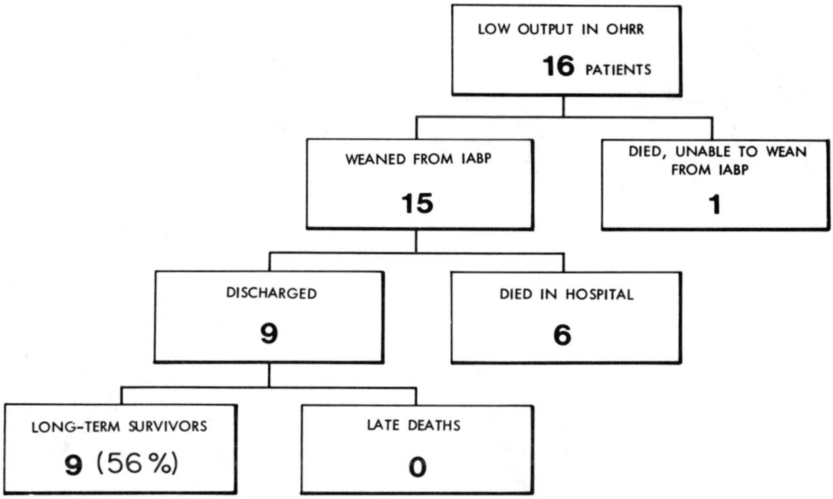

FIG. 12. Postoperative unidirectional intra-aortic balloon pumping (IABP), Columbia Presbyterian Medical Center, 1972–76: Group C. OHRR, open heart recovery room.

monary bypass and the initial graft blood flow was measured during IABP, repeat measurements were also performed with the patient on and off assistance just prior to closure of the chest. These changes in coronary blood flow, which can be attributed to the balloon alone, demonstrated an average increase of 83 percent (range, 40 to 100 percent; median, 80 percent). The increase in coronary blood flow was sustained during a 2-minute period of observation. Examples of the improvement in coronary blood flow with unidirectional IABP can be seen in Figure 11.

Group C: This group consisted of 16 patients who were assisted an average of 13 hours after the completion of open heart surgery (Fig. 12). The duration of IABP averaged 60 hours, an increase of 33 percent in time over the assist period for group B patients. With the onset of IABP, the left atrial pressures fell an average of 13 mm Hg, and the central venous pressures fell an average of 7 cm of water in those patients who responded to the assist. Mean arterial blood pressure rose 36 mm Hg. Urinary outputs increased an average of 36 cc per hour in the first hour of IABP. As in the other patient groups, there was a marked decrease in the concurrent requirement for inotropic support. Of the sixteen patients in this category, 13 had a significant intra-

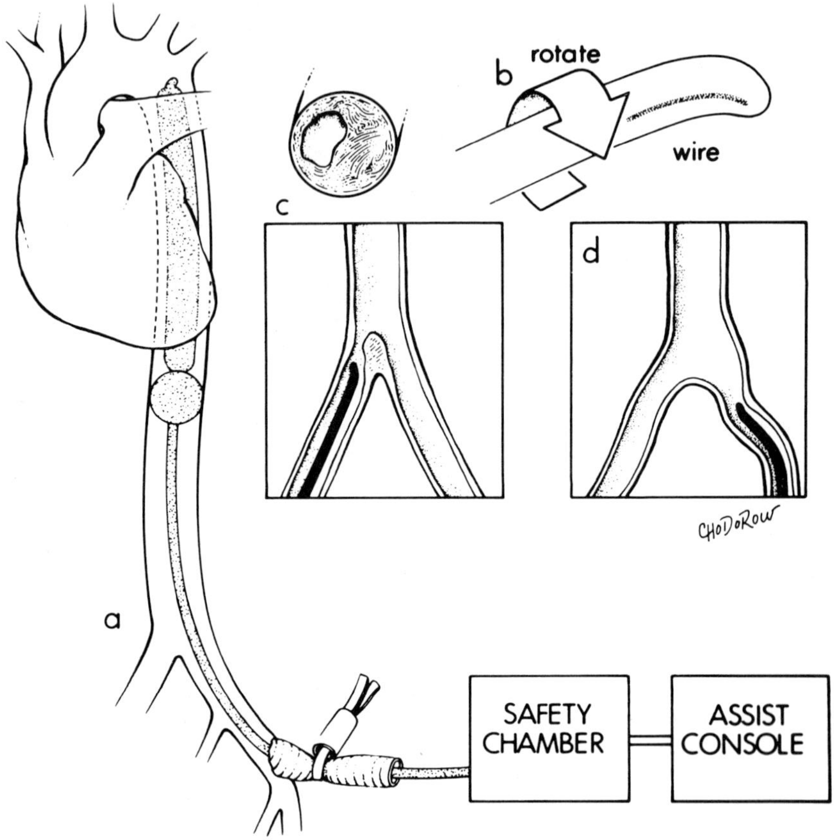

FIG. 13. (a) Proper position of dual-chambered intra-aortic balloon just distal to left subclavian artery. Note that the balloon is inserted through a Dacron prosthesis which is snared, permitting perfusion of the distal extremity during the period of cardiac assist. (b) Technique of bending and rotating distal balloon catheter during insertion. (c) Balloon negotiating eccentric arteriosclerotic stenosis. (d) Balloon passing through an arterial tortuosity.

operative acute myocardial infarction, and all of the patients undergoing coronary revascularization had at least one coronary graft in which the intraoperative blood flow measurement at the conclusion of cardiopulmonary bypass was less than 25 cc per minute. The changes in the course of these patients with acute myocardial ischemia and its complications suggest that such patients can obtain the maximum beneficial response to IABP only if a careful early protocol is adapted, so that the greatest mass of is-

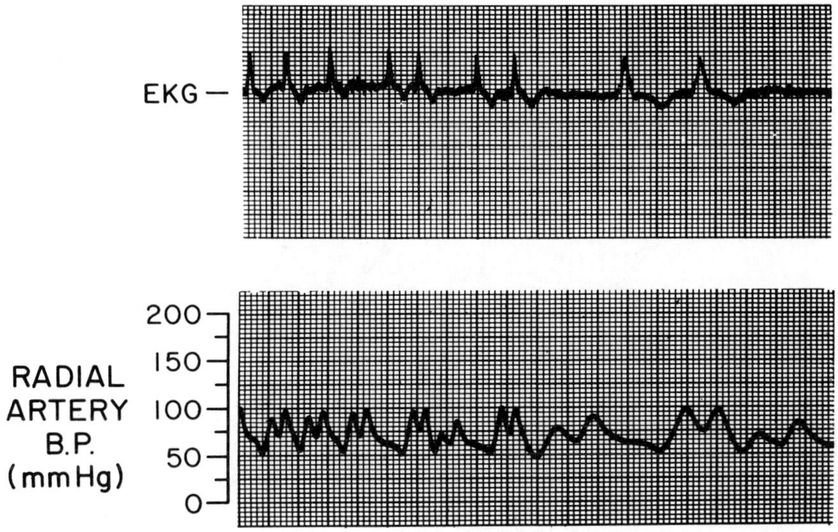

FIG. 14. Patient with atrial fibrillation undergoing IABP. Note automatic variation of diastolic interval during synchronous 1:1 assist.

chemic myocardium will be preserved. Of the 16 patients assisted in this group, 15 could be weaned from intra-aortic balloon pumping, and 9 patients or 56 percent were discharged from the hospital.

COMPLICATIONS

Complications of intra-aortic balloon pumping in the present series were relatively few. The balloon could not be inserted in one patient who would have been included in the group A category. In 18 patients, however, the balloon tip required bending (Fig. 13) so that it could be inserted in the ipsilateral extremity.[12] In one group B patient in whom the balloon could not be inserted in either extremity, the balloon was inserted directly in the ascending aorta.[13] This patient was successfully weaned from cardiopulmonary bypass and was returned to the operating room three days later for opening of the chest and removal of the balloon. Relative limb ischema, which abated after 1 hour, was seen in four patients. There were no late peripheral vascular complications. In addition, there were no local infections, and two lymph fistulas closed spontaneously within two months. None of the patients undergoing valve replacement were noted to develop sepsis. No patient had demonstrable emboli, and arrhythmias were tracked without incident (Fig. 14).

Table 1 outlines the clinical summary for all 63 patients undergoing IABP.

TABLE 1. Columbia-Presbyterian Medical Center: Unidirectional Intra-Aortic Balloon Pumping and Open Heart Surgery*

Total patients	63
Number weaned from IABP	55 (87%)
Number discharged	40 (63%)

**Data collected from Feb. 1, 1972, through April 30, 1976.*

THE PULSATILE ASSIST DEVICE (PAD)

Although the advantages of pulsatile cardiopulmonary bypass have been well documented,[14–22]

1. Better capillary perfusion
2. Less metabolic acidosis
3. Increased oxygen consumption
4. Lower peripheral arterial resistance
5. Better renal perfusion
6. Improved cerebral perfusion
7. Less hepatocellular injury
8. Better myocardial perfusion (especially in the subendocardium)
9. Less elevation of coronary sinus lactate

it has, up until now, not been possible to routinely use pulsation during open heart surgery. Evidence from Berger[23] and Pappas[24] has clearly documented the advantages of pulsatile cardiopulmonary bypass when an intra-aortic balloon pump was used to create the pulsations.

A new pulsatile assist device (PAD) has been developed to convert in a simple fashion roller pump flow to pulsatile flow

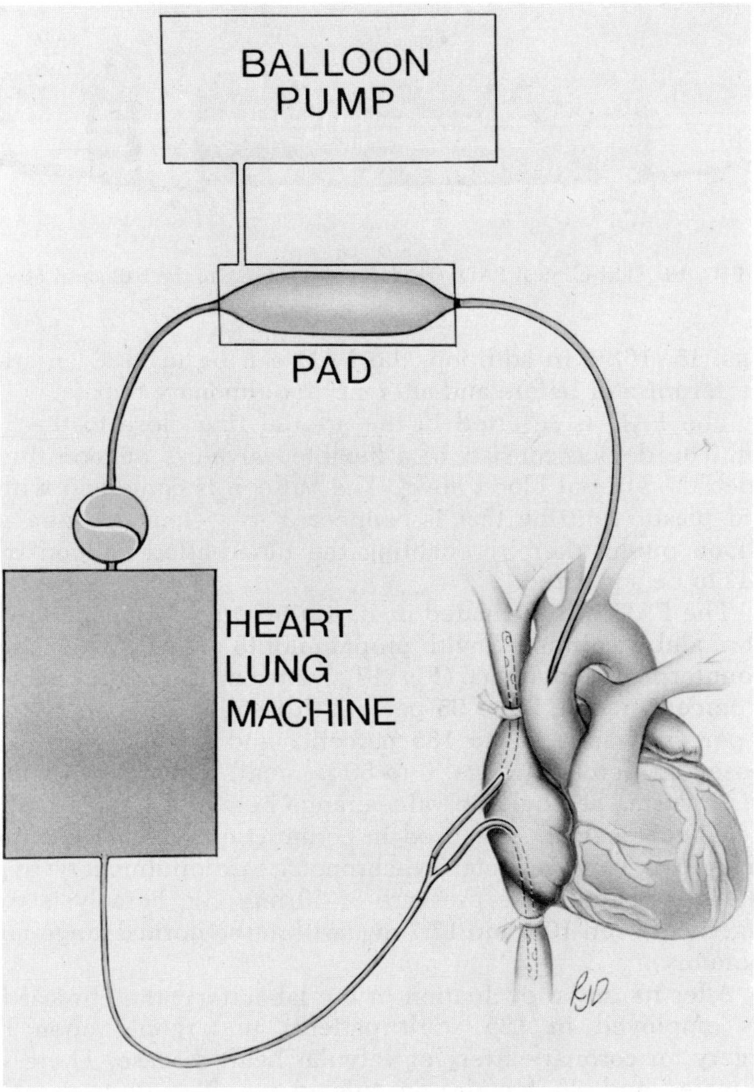

FIG. 15. Schematic of Pulsatile Assist Device (PAD) in cardiopulmonary bypass circuit. Oxygenated blood flows through the valveless balloon within the PAD, and then into the aorta. The balloon pump pneumatically squeezes the PAD balloon to effect either synchronous counterpulsation or pulsatile cardiopulmonary bypass.

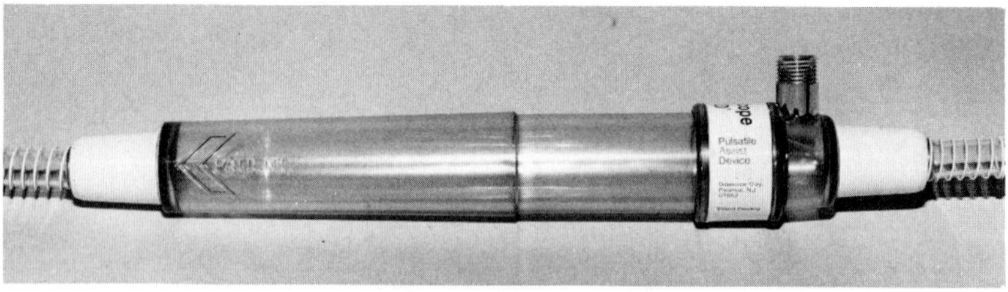

FIG. 16. The clinical PAD. Displacement volume of the balloon is 80 cc.

(Figs. 15, 16).[25] In addition, the PAD can be used as an arterial counterpulsater before and after cardiopulmonary bypass.

The PAD is inserted in the arterial line close to the aortic root. The device consists of a flexible valveless balloon through which the arterial blood flows. The balloon is contained within a rigid plastic housing that is connected to a standard intra-aortic balloon pump, thereby enabling the blood-filled balloon in the PAD to be squeezed.

The PAD was evaluated in 12 canine preparations. A low output model was induced with propranolol (3 mg/kg). When used as a counterpulsation device (Fig. 17), mean cardiac output increased 53 percent (range, 25 to 95 percent), diastolic pressure increased 99 percent (range, 33 to 165 percent), and systolic pressure decreased 12 percent (range, 0 to 50 percent). During two hours of assist, plasma hemoglobin values range between 4 and 12 mg.[26]

When the PAD was used in conjunction with a roller pump during two hours of total synchronous cardiopulmonary bypass, with an average pulse pressure of 40 mm Hg, hemolysis values ranged between 10.5 and 17.7 mg (within the normal range for our laboratory).

After its initial evaluation in the laboratory, the clinical PAD was employed in 125 adult patients undergoing open heart surgery for coronary artery or valvular heart disease. There were 99 males and 26 females in this group. Twenty-two patients underwent isolated valve replacement, five had resection of a ventricular aneurysm alone, eight patients underwent combined ventricular aneurysm resection with coronary artery revascularization, thirteen patients underwent combined valve replacement and coronary revascularization, and seventy-seven patients underwent coronary artery revascularization alone. Ninety-two patients in this

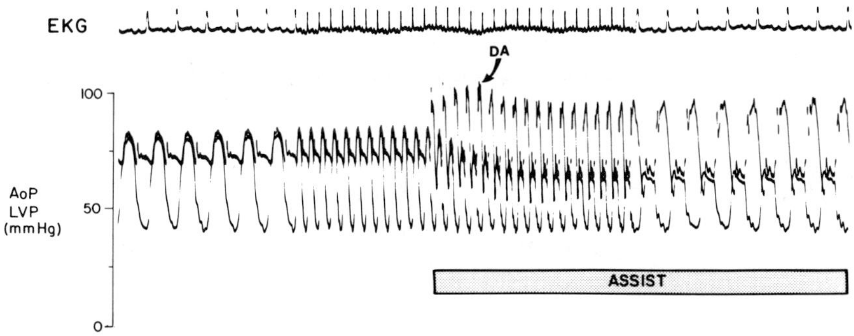

FIG. 17. Effect of the PAD is an arterial counterpulsator. Note significant pressure (unloading) and large diastolic augmentation during the assist. Tracing speed, 25 mm/sec; EKG, electrocardiogram; AoP, aortic pressure; LVP, left ventricular pressure; DA, diastolic augmentation.

group were either New York Heart Association class III or IV, or had ejection fractions of less than 0.3. In the clinical setting, the device functioned as a hemodynamically effective counterpulsator both before and after cardiopulmonary bypass. During bypass, pulse pressures of 40 to 50 mm Hg were readily obtained (Fig. 18). Urinary outputs during cardiopulmonary bypass were increased with the PAD when compared to a control group (9.18 ± .68 cc per minute versus 3.90 ± .35 cc per minute). In addition, during cardiopulmonary bypass, coronary graft blood flow increased an average of 21.4 percent with the PAD, and after cardiopulmonary bypass, coronary blood flow increased an average of 25.0 percent. Free plasma hemoglobins after cardiopulmonary bypass were not elevated when compared to a control group.

CLINICAL RESULTS WITH THE PAD

In the group of 125 patients assisted with the PAD, all patients were successfully weaned from cardiopulmonary bypass with the PAD alone. In one patient, it was necessary to insert an intra-aortic balloon postoperatively. This patient incurred an acute intraoperative myocardial infarction, the only patient who experienced such an infarction in the 125 patients. His postoperative course with intra-aortic balloon pumping was uneventful. One additional patient, who was successfully operated upon in conjunc-

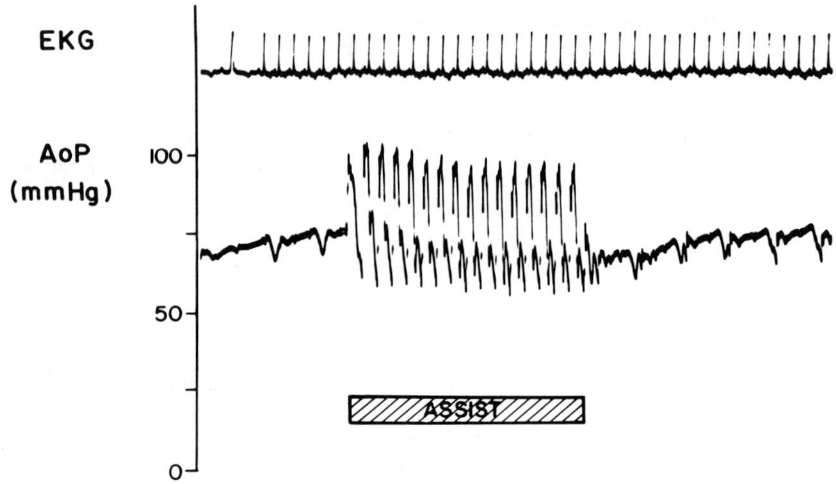

FIG. 18. Effect of the PAD to create synchronous pulsatile cardiopulmonary bypass. Note pulse pressure of 45 mm Hg during bypass. EKG, electrocardiogram; AoP, aortic pressure.

tion with the PAD, expired in the recovery room from an anaphylactic reaction to a drug. There were 3 late deaths. Suggested criteria for PAD use are as follow:

1. Preoperative NYHA Class III or IV
2. Preoperative ejection fraction $< .3$
3. Preoperative LVEDP $\geqslant$ 18 mm Hg
4. Patients with left main Coronary Artery Lesions or equivalent left main lesions
5. Patients with Crescendo Angina refractory to medical therapy who have previously been studied
6. Patients requiring an Aortic Valve Replacement in conjunction with Coronary Artery Bypass surgery
7. Patients in whom the CPB is expected to be $>$ 3 hours

NEW BALLOONS

Pediatric IABP

A pediatric single-chambered balloon has been developed on a special catheter (Fig. 19).[2] This balloon has been utilized in two patients with a low cardiac output syndrome at the Columbia Presbyterian Medical Center. In one infant patient, the balloon

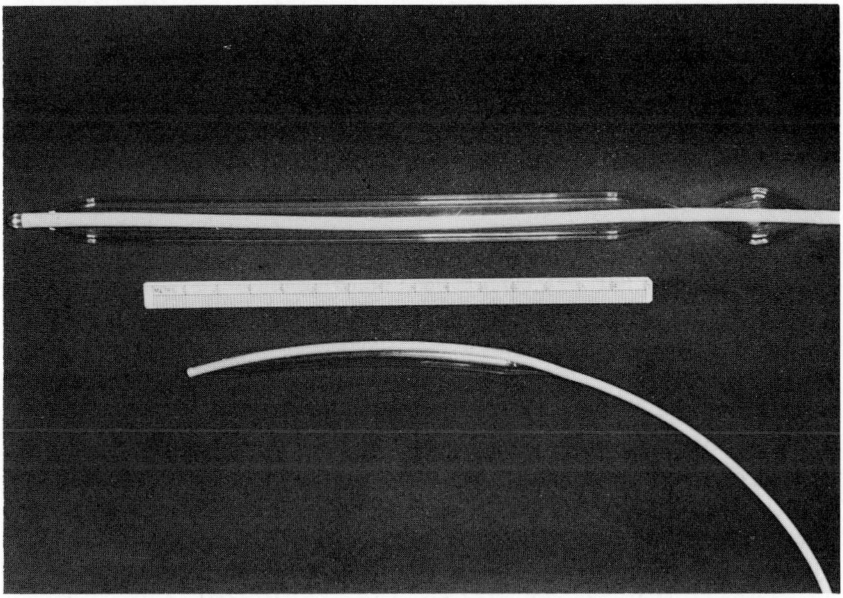

FIG. 19. Pediatric balloon compared with adult intra-aortic balloon.

was inserted directly in the ascending aorta. This patient was more than 48 hours postoperatively, and although he initially responded to the balloon pump, he ultimately expired. A second 12-year-old patient was assisted 48 hours postoperatively for a low cardiac output syndrome after a complex repair of a tetralogy of Fallot. This patient survived after 48 hours of balloon assist.

Left Ventricular Balloon Pumping

In the experimental low cardiac output state, intra-aortic balloon pumping may be hemodynamically ineffective if the initial systolic blood pressure is less than 45 mm Hg. In this instance, a more direct left ventricular assist device may be required. A left ventricular balloon has been developed which can be inserted directly into the left ventricular cavity through the apex of the left ventricle. The balloon is inflated during systole, thereby directly propelling blood out of the left ventricle and into the aorta. The left ventricular balloon has been shown to be an extremely effective cardiac assist device in the experimental low output setting

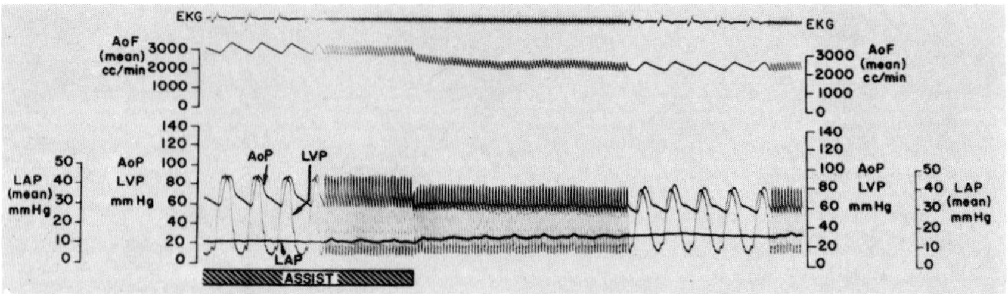

FIG. 20. Effect of left ventricular balloon pumping in canine cardiogenic shock. Note that when the assist is discontinued, there is a fall in aortic flow (AoF), aortic pressure (AoP), and left ventricular pressure (LVP), with a rise in left atrial pressure (LAP).

(Fig. 20) by its ability to cause a rapid fall in left atrial pressure and in left ventricular end diastolic pressure with concurrent improvement in aortic pressure, aortic flow, and in coronary blood flow.[27] A pear-shaped model for clinical use is now available (Fig. 21). It is felt that the left ventricular balloon may predispose to the development of subendocardial ischemia. It is therefore recommended that in the clinical setting this balloon be used in conjunction with an intra-aortic balloon in the same patient. The increase in wall tension caused by the left ventricular balloon is more than offset by the improvement in the transmural myocardial blood flow from the concurrent use of the intra-aortic balloon pump.

DISCUSSION

Although intra-aortic balloon pumping has been employed experimentally for the past sixteen years[28] and clinically for the past eight years,[29] only recently have clinical data become available to evaluate its use in a variety of clinical settings. Initially, it was felt that intervention with intra-aortic balloon pumping in a patient with acute myocardial infarction and cardiogenic shock would lead to increased patient survival. However, although the shock syndrome is frequently reversed, the ultimate outcome has not been significantly altered.[30]

The most successful use of intra-aortic balloon pumping to date has been as an adjunct to the pre-, intra-, and postoperative support of patients undergoing open heart surgery.[1,30] As can be seen in our group A patients, it is now possible to stabilize the

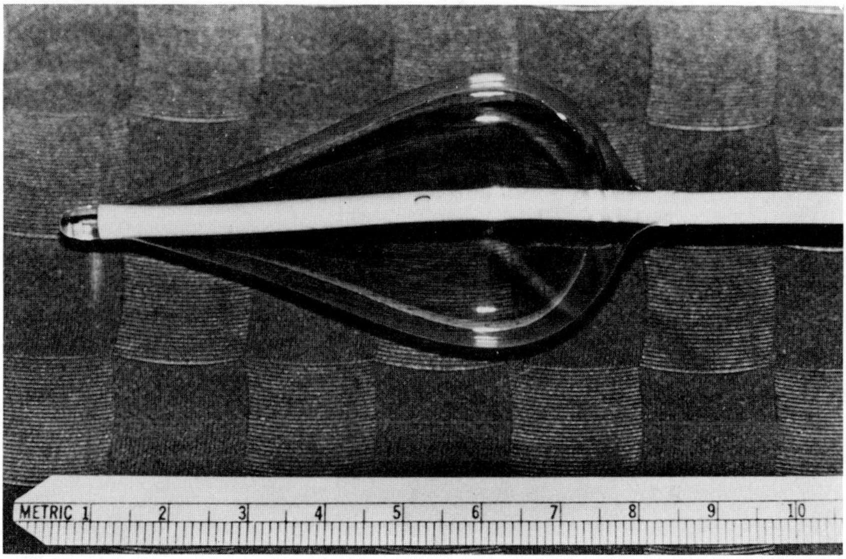

FIG. 21. The clinical pear-shaped left ventricular balloon.

condition of critically ill individuals, subject them to cardiac catheterization safely, and bring them to the operating room in a more stable condition. Patients with hepatic and renal failure secondary to their cardiac lesion can be markedly improved with intra-aortic balloon pumping prior to surgery. Also, high-risk patients and those individuals with critical coronary artery lesions can undergo anesthetic induction in a relatively safe fashion with intra-aortic balloon support until cardiopulmonary bypass can be safely established. The results in our group B and C patients demonstrate the success of intra-aortic balloon pumping in its role in weaning patients from cardiopulmonary bypass who have incurred either subendocardial ischemia or infarction during the procedure, and in supporting them in the postoperative period.

Our clinical data confirms the theoretical and experimental observations of Buckberg and associates,[10] who suggested that the adequacy of subendocardial perfusion and potential ischemia could be predicted from indices derived from systolic and diastolic pressure measurements. Since ischemia appears to be the most common cause of the low cardiac output syndrome following open heart surgery, it is imperative to recognize the condition early if proper therapy is to be initiated in time to prevent myocardial necrosis.

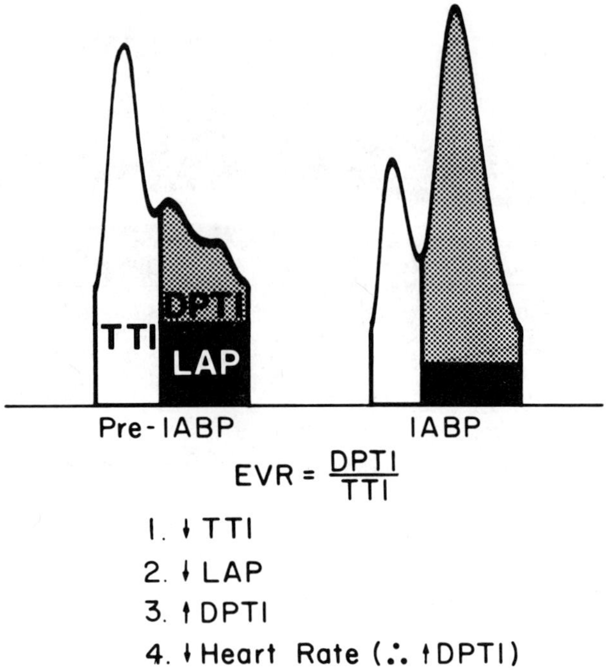

FIG. 22. Effects of unidirectional intra-aortic balloon pumping on the endocardial viability ratio (EVR). DPTI, diastolic pressure-time index; TTI, tension-time index; LAP, left atrial pressure.

The concept of the EVR appears particularly well suited for use in monitoring patients undergoing unidirectional IABP, because there are at least four favorable alterations that the balloon imposes on this ratio (Fig. 22).[31] First, the area under the systolic pressure curve falls with balloon pumping. This is a reflection of the decrease in the impedance to left ventricular ejection caused by proper balloon deflation during intra-aortic balloon pumping. The TTI is decreased, and therefore the EVR will increase. Second, the left atrial pressure falls during IABP, and thus the resting left ventricular wall tension decreases. Third, the area under the diastolic pressure curve will markedly rise during unidirectional IABP, which will increase myocardial oxygen supply or the DPTI. Finally, the heart rate will be slowed by reflex and other mechanisms, an effect that will primarily lengthen the diastolic period and also increase the EVR.

The increase in coronary blood flow during intra-aortic bal-

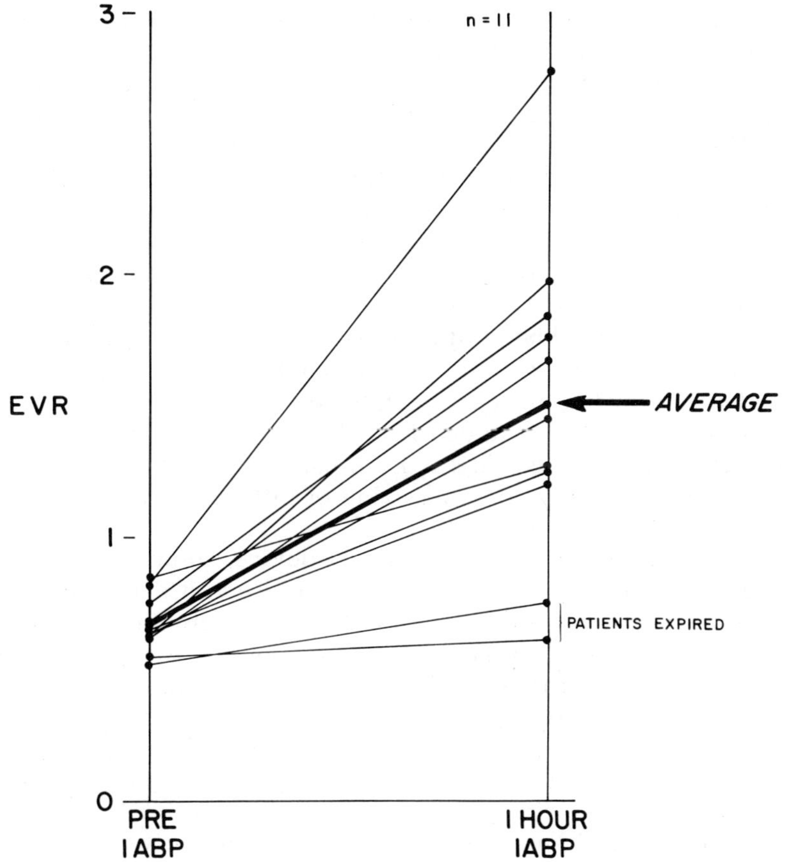

FIG. 23. Effects of unidirectional intra-aortic balloon pumping (IABP) on the endocardial viability ratio (EVR) in 11 group B patients.

loon pumping, documented in our patients, in conjunction with the improvement in EVR (Fig. 23), suggests that a redistribution of transmural coronary blood flow has occurred and that the previously jeopardized subendocardial muscle is now being adequately perfused. The hospital survival (87 percent) and the long-term survival (63 percent) rates in our series compares well with the encouraging data reported by other groups in similar patients.[32–45]

An analysis of the data obtained in patients assisted with unidirectional IABP in conjunction with open heart surgery at the Columbia Presbyterian Medical Center has led to two groups of criteria for employing intraoperative IABP.[1]

The primary indications for intraoperative IABP as suggested by our data include any two of criteria 1 to 3, in conjunction with criteria 4, in patients in whom weaning from cardiopulmonary bypass has been attempted for 1 hour: (a) mean blood pressure, 60 mm Hg and falling; (b) cardiac index, 1.8 liters per minute per square meter and falling; (c) left atrial pressure, 25 mm Hg and rising; and (d) requirement for high-dose inotropic support.

Additional criteria include the following: (a) recurrent ventricular tachyarrhythmias; (b) evidence of a significant intraoperative myocardial infarction; (c) subendocardial ischemia (EVR less than 0.8 at the conclusion of bypass); and (d) coronary graft blood flow less than 40 cc per minute (projected use).

It is interesting, in retrospect, to see that most of our group C patients fell into these categories. They would now probably become group B patients. This will be particularly true when better methods for the detection and sizing of intraoperative myocardial infarcts become available.

With regard to the pulsatile assist device, certain conclusions can be drawn from our initial experience. First, it is now possible to utilize counterpulsation routinely and safely in open heart surgery. The pulsatile assist device functions in every respect as an intraoperative intra-aortic balloon pump, without the need for additional surgery. It has been interesting to see that in our initial evaluation of the pulsatile assist device, the advantages of pulsatile cardiopulmonary bypass are being supported and clarified. Certainly, greater urinary output indirectly implies better renal perfusion. In addition, the increase in intraoperative myocardial blood flow would appear to offer greater protection to the myocardium during cardiopulmonary bypass. The extremely low incidence of perioperative myocardial infarctions in this series would attest to this fact. Of more interest is the fact that during our initial six-month clinical utilization of the pulsatile assist device, only one patient required intraoperative intra-aortic balloon pumping. This is a marked reduction in the requirement for balloon pumping at our institution and suggests that the use of the pulsatile assist device will probably decrease the need for postoperative intra-aortic balloon pumping.

It is concluded that the primary use for intra-aortic balloon pumping is currently assistance of the open heart surgical patient (Fig. 24). The criteria are now defined. It is our impression that the use of intra-aortic balloon pumping in selected patients undergoing open heart surgery has lead to improved patient survival

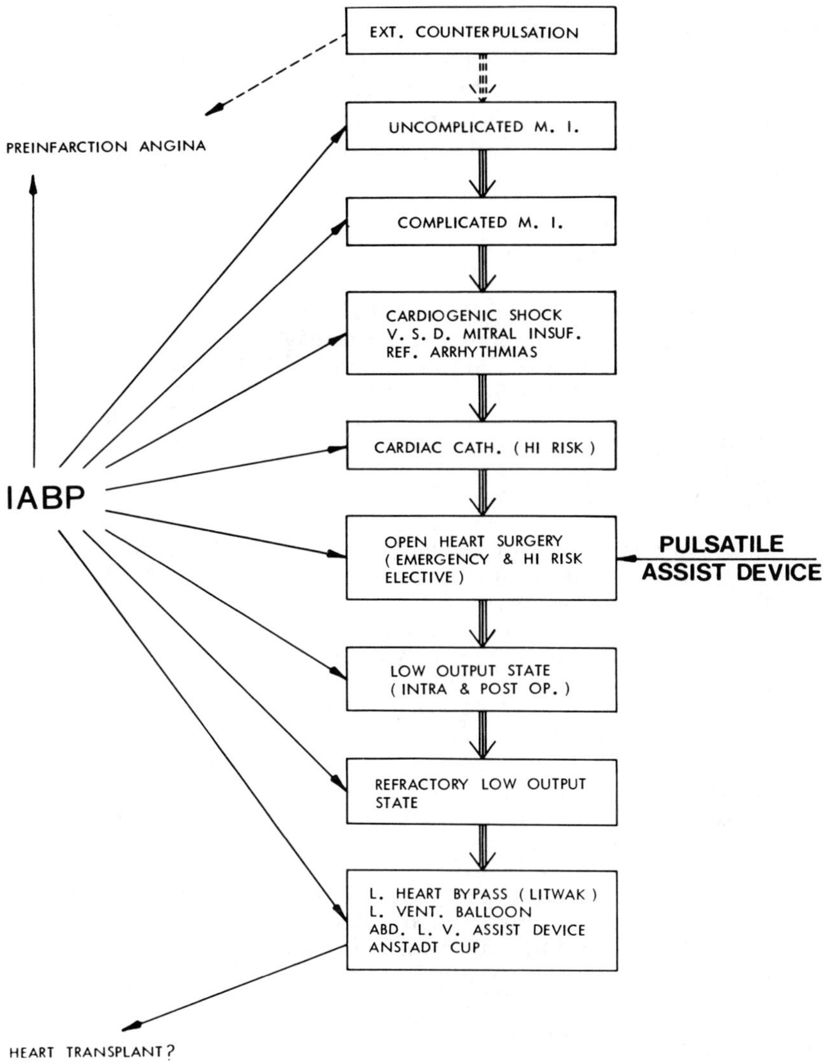

FIG. 24. The role of left heart assist devices in clinical medicine.

and has enabled us to operate upon high-risk patients with greater confidence and with improved clinical results. More significantly, use of the pulsatile assist device will extend the role of counterpulsation in open heart surgery and will probably decrease the need for postoperative balloon pumping in these high-risk patients.

REFERENCES

1. Bregman D, Parodi EN, Edie RN, et al: Intraoperative unidirectional intra-aortic balloon pumping in the management of left ventricular power failure. J Thorac Cardiovasc Surg 70:1010, 1975
2. Bregman D, Parodi EN, Reemtsma K, Malm JR: Advances in clinical intraaortic balloon pumping. In Norman JC (ed): Coronary Artery Medicine and Surgery: Concepts and Controversies. New York, Appleton, 1975, pp 413–20
3. Najafi H, Henson D, Dye WS et al: Left ventricular hemorrhagic necrosis. Ann Thorac Surg 7:550, 1969
4. Buckberg GD, Towers B, Paglia DE, Mulder DG, Maloney JS: Subendocardial ischemia after cardiopulmonary bypass. J Thorac Cardiovasc Surg 64:669, 1972
5. Bregman D, Goetz RH: A failsafe cardiac assist system for intraaortic balloon pumping. Trans Am Soc Artif Intern Organs 18:505, 1972
6. Bregman D, Kripke DC, Goetz RH: The effect of synchronous unidirectional intra-aortic balloon pumping on hemodynamics and coronary blood flow in cardiogenic shock. Trans Am Soc Artif Intern Organs 16:439, 1970
7. Bregman D, Goetz RH: Clinical experience with a new cardiac assist device: The dual-chambered intra-aortic balloon assist. J Thorac Cardiovasc Surg 62:577, 1971
8. Bregman D: Management of patients undergoing intra-aortic balloon pumping. Heart and Lung 3:916, 1974
9. Weisel RD, Berger RL, Hechtman HB: Measurement of cardiac output by thermodilution. N Eng J Med 292:682, 1975
10. Buckberg GD, Fixler DE, Archie JP, Hoffman JIE: Experimental subendocardial ischemia in dogs with normal coronary arteries. Circ Res 30:67, 1972
11. Philips PA, Marty AT, Miyamoto AM: A clinical method for detecting subendocardial ischemia after cardiopulmonary bypass. J Thorac Cardiovasc Surg 69:30, 1975
12. Bregman D, Bolooki H, Malm JR: A simple method to facilitate difficult intra-aortic balloon insertions. Ann Thorac Surg 15:636, 1973
13. Printup CA, Dietrick WR, Getzen JH, et al: Ascending aorta insertion of the dual-chambered intra-aortic balloon for counterpulsation during cardiac operations. Ann Thorac Surg 20:694, 1975

14. Boucher JK, Rudy LW, Jr, Edmunds LH, Jr: Organ blood flow during pulsatile cardiopulmonary bypass. J Appl Physiol 36:86, 1974
15. Dunn J, Kirsh MM, Harness J, et al: Hemodynamic, metabolic, and hematologic effects of pulsatile cardiopulmonary bypass. J Thorac Cardiovasc Surg 68:138, 1974
16. Habal SM, Weiss MB, Spotnitz HM, et al: Effects of pulsatile and nonpulsatile coronary perfusion on canine left ventricular performance. J Thorac Cardiovasc Surg 72:742, 1976
17. Hewitt RL, Weichert RF: Diastolic augmentation during heart bypass. J Thorac Cardiovasc Surg 60:123, 1970
18. Jacobs LA, Klopp EH, Seamone W, Topaz SR, Gott VL: Improved organ function during cardiac bypass with a roller pump modified to deliver pulsatile flow. J Thorac Cardiovasc Surg 58:703, 1969
19. Morkin E: Analysis of pulsatile blood flow and its clinical implications. New Eng J Med 277:139, 1967
20. Trinkle JK, Helton NE, Wood RE, Bryant LR: Metabolic comparison of a new pulsatile pump and a roller pump for cardiopulmonary bypass. J Thorac Cardiovasc Surg 58:562, 1969
21. Trinkle JK, Helton NE, Bryant LR, Griffen WO: Pulsatile cardiopulmonary bypass: Clinical evaluation. Surgery 68:1074, 1970
22. Wright G, Sanderson JM: Brain damage and mortality in dogs following pulsatile and nonpulsatile blood flows in extracorporeal circulation. Thorax 27:738, 1972
23. Berger RL, Saini VK: Conversion of nonpulsatile cardiopulmonary bypass to pulsatile flow by intra-aortic balloon pumping during myocardial revascularization for cardiogenic shock (abstract). Circulation XLV and XLVI:130, 1972 (suppl II)
24. Pappas G, Winter SD, Kopriva CJ, Steele PP: Improvement of myocardial and other vital organ functions and metabolism with a simple method of pulsatile flow (IABP) during clinical cardiopulmonary bypass. Surgery 77:34, 1975
25. Bregman D, Parodi EN, Bowman FO, Jr, et al: Clinical experience with a new cardiac assist device—the pulsatile assist device (PAD) (abstract). Clinical Res 24:211A, 1976
26. Habal S, Parodi EN, Hanson B, Wolvek S, Bregman D: A new pulsatile assist device (PAD) for use in cardiac surgery. Abstracts ASA10 5:32, 1976
27. Bregman D, Parodi EN, Malm JR: Left ventricular unidirectional intra-aortic balloon pumping. J Thorac Cardiovasc Surg 68:677, 1974
28. Moulopoulos SD, Topaz S, Kolff WJ: Diastolic balloon pumping (with carbon dioxide) in the aorta: A mechanical assistance to the failing circulation. Am Heart J 63:669, 1962
29. Kantrowitz A, Tjønneland S, Freed PS, et al: Initial clinical experience with intra-aortic balloon pumping in cardiogenic shock. JAMA 203:113, 1968
30. Bregman D: Assessment of intra-aortic balloon counterpulsation in cardiogenic shock. J Crit Care Med 3:90, 1975
31. Bregman D: Discussion of Philips et al[11]
32. Baron DW, O'Rourke MF: Long-term results of arterial counterpul-

sation in acute severe cardiac failure complicating myocardial infarction. Brit Heart J 38:285, 1976

33. Bolooki H, Williams W, Thurer RJ, et al: Clinical and hemodynamic criteria for use of the intra-aortic balloon pump (IABP) in cardiac surgery patients. J Thorac Cardiovasc Surg 72:46, 1976
34. Burman SO: Intra-aortic balloon pumping for low cardiac output syndromes. Surg Clin No Amer 55:101, 1975
35. Cleveland JC, Lefemine AA, Madoff I, et al: The role of intra-aortic balloon counterpulsation in patients undergoing cardiac operations. Ann Thorac Surg 20:652, 1975
36. Cohn L: Intra-aortic balloon counterpulsation in low cardiac output states. Surg Clin No Amer 55:545, 1975
37. Foster ED, Subramanian VA, Vito L, Hechtman HB, Berger RL: Response to intra-aortic balloon pumping. Am J Surg 129:464, 1975
38. Goldman BS, Gunstensen J, Gilbert BW, et al: Increasing operability and survival with intra-aortic balloon pump assist. Canad J Surg 19:69, 1976
39. Housman LB, Casey C, Speros D, et al: Intra-aortic balloon counterpulsation in the treatment of refractory intra-operative cardiogenic shock. J Extra-Corp Tech VII:84, 1975
40. Lamberti JJ, Anagnostopoulos CE, Al-Sadir J, et al: Mechanical circulatory assistance for the treatment of complications of coronary artery disease. Surg Clin No Amer 56:83, 1976
41. Mundth ED: Mechanical and surgical interventions for the reduction of myocardial ischemia. Circulation 53:I-176, 1976
42. O'Donovan TG: The use of intra-aortic balloon pumping in cardiac surgical patients. S A Med J 50:74, 1976
43. Webb WR, Parker FB, Neville JF, Hanson EL: Acute mechanical complications of coronary arterial disease. Arch Surg 109:251, 1974
44. Weintraub RM, Voukydis PC, Aroesty JM, et al: Treatment of preinfarction angina with intra-aortic balloon counterpulsation and surgery. Am J Card 34:809, 1974
45. Willerson JT, Curry GC, Watson JT, et al: Intra-aortic balloon counterpulsation in patients in cardiogenic shock, medically refractory left ventricular failure and/or recurrent ventricular tachycardia. Am J Med 58:183, 1975

CHAPTER 3

Management of Low Cardiac Output after Open Intracardiac Operation with a Left Heart Assist Device

Robert S. Litwak
Robert M. Koffsky
Roy A. Jurado
Salvador B. Lukban
Arcadio F. Ortiz
Vincente Grana
Adam Fischer
James J. Sherman
George Silvay
Fouad A. Lajam
Richard A. deAsla
Hillard L. Fitzkee

It is remarkable that despite the widening spectrum and increasing complexity of open intracardiac operations, mortality is low in patients coming to surgery with adequate cardiac performance. However, hospital mortality is substantially higher in those patients entering the operating room with advanced cardiac dysfunction. Although methods of quantitating cardiac performance are still relatively crude, an ejection fraction of less than 0.3[1–4] (Table 1) or a cardiac index less than 1.7 to 1.9[5–6] in a potential surgical candidate convey a heightened probability that life-threatening low cardiac output may occur either in the operating room or during the early postoperative period. It is apparent that simple and effective methods of temporary left heart support could be lifesaving in such patients. Afterload reduction, employing intra-aortic balloon counterpulsation (IABC) has been demonstrably effective in salvaging many patients whose cardiac performance was insufficient to allow them to be separated from conventional cardiopulmonary bypass at the conclusion of the intracardiac procedure.[7–10]

TABLE 1. Relationship of Ventricular Ejection Fraction and Surgical Mortality

SOURCE OF DATA	EJECTION FRACTION	SURGICAL MORTALITY (PERCENT)
Oldham et al[1]	≤.25	55
	>.25	4
Lea et al[2]	≤.25	51
	.46–.50	11
Hammermeister and Kennedy[3]	≤.33	33
	>.33	3.1
Cohn et al[4]	<.50	35
	≥.50	3

Despite the unquestioned efficacy of IABC, there remains a small cohort of patients who, if they are to survive, must be provided with a mechanical means of supporting a substantial amount of total systemic blood flow (TSBF) requirements until their hearts recover from the operative trauma sufficiently to again sustain life. It is the purpose of this report to describe our efforts to both reduce left ventricular (LV) preload and augment TSBF utilizing a simple left heart assist device (LHAD).

CONCEPTS OF THE LHAD

Clinical Background

Virtually all cardiac surgeons have had the frustrating experience of being able to temporarily stabilize the hemodynamic state of a patient after intracardiac repair as long as 25 to 50 percent of the calculated TSBF was shunted around the left ventricle but, on the other hand, not being able to discontinue that level of support because of persistently poor cardiac function. If all intraoperative supportive measures ultimately proved inadequate, there was no course open other than to decide when to turn off the extracorporeal pump-oxygenator.

LHAD Design

In view of the observation that partial LV bypass could temporarily stabilize the patient in the operating room, a method of accomplishing this was sought which would permit circulatory support for periods as long as one month, the hypothesis being that preload reduction would establish conditions favoring cardiac recovery while TSBF was mechanically maintained at adequate levels. Following several years of experimental work[11] a LHAD was developed, the details of which have been described in previous communications.[12,13] Briefly, the LHAD simply consists of silicone elastomer cannulae with polyester sewing skirts* (Fig. 1), which allow convenient suturing to the left atrium (LA) and ascending aorta; an extracorporeal tubing loop and roller pump complete the circuit (Fig. 2). The current system permits left heart support flows up to 5 liters per minute. The distal tips of the LHAD cannulae lie subcutaneously in the right upper quadrant of the abdomen. When LHAD support is ultimately discontinued, the distal cannula tips are easily exposed; a precisely fitting obturator is inserted into each cannula, which thereby obliterates the luminal dead space while creating smooth planar surfaces at the LA and aortic cannulation sites. Thus, LHAD separation is accomplished without need for thoracic reentry. Since the cannula

**Components available from Hancock Laboratories Inc., 4633 E. LaPalma Avenue, Anaheim, California.*

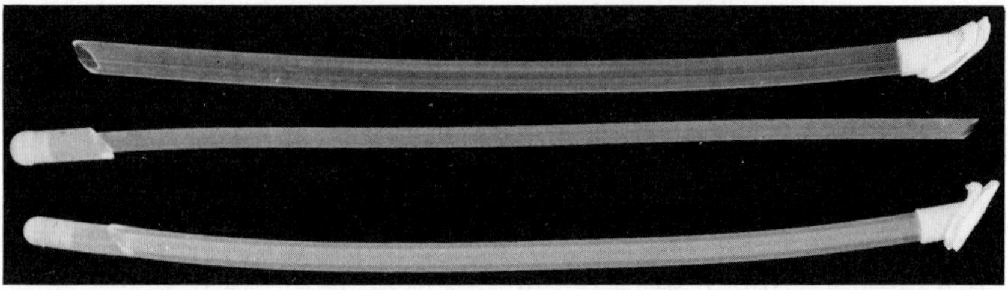

FIG. 1. The cannula and obturator design. The proximal cannula tips are angulated to conform to the anatomical relationships of the left atrium and ascending aorta. Hemostatic suturing is facilitated by double polyester skirts. When circulatory support is discontinued, an obturator (middle) is inserted into the cannula lumen so that the luminal space is obliterated (bottom). Proper orientation of the obturator within the cannula is assured by the matching angularity of the obturator shoulder and the distal cannula tip. (From Litwak et al: Ann Thorac Surg 21:191, 1976)

and obturator components are fabricated from materials of established long-term biocompatibility in man, they are permitted to remain permanently in situ (Fig. 3).

EMPLOYMENT OF THE LHAD

The Decision to Deploy the LHAD

As suggested earlier, the LHAD is used only as a last resort after prolonged use (1 to 2 hours) of all supportive measures (including use of IABC whenever possible) have failed to permit discontinuance of conventional cardiopulmonary bypass. Criteria of life-threatening cardiac depression which must persist during the attempted bypass weaning process include elevated LV filling pressure (mean LA pressure greater than 25 mm Hg) in the presence of systemic hypotension (peak systolic pressure less than 90 mm Hg), and visibly poor LV contractility.

Deployment and Operation of the LHAD

After suturing the cannulae into place, they are connected to the extracorporeal tubing loop and roller pump. Since the LA and aortic cannulae will remain in situ after use, it is essential that they lie totally intracorporeal and never traverse the skin in order

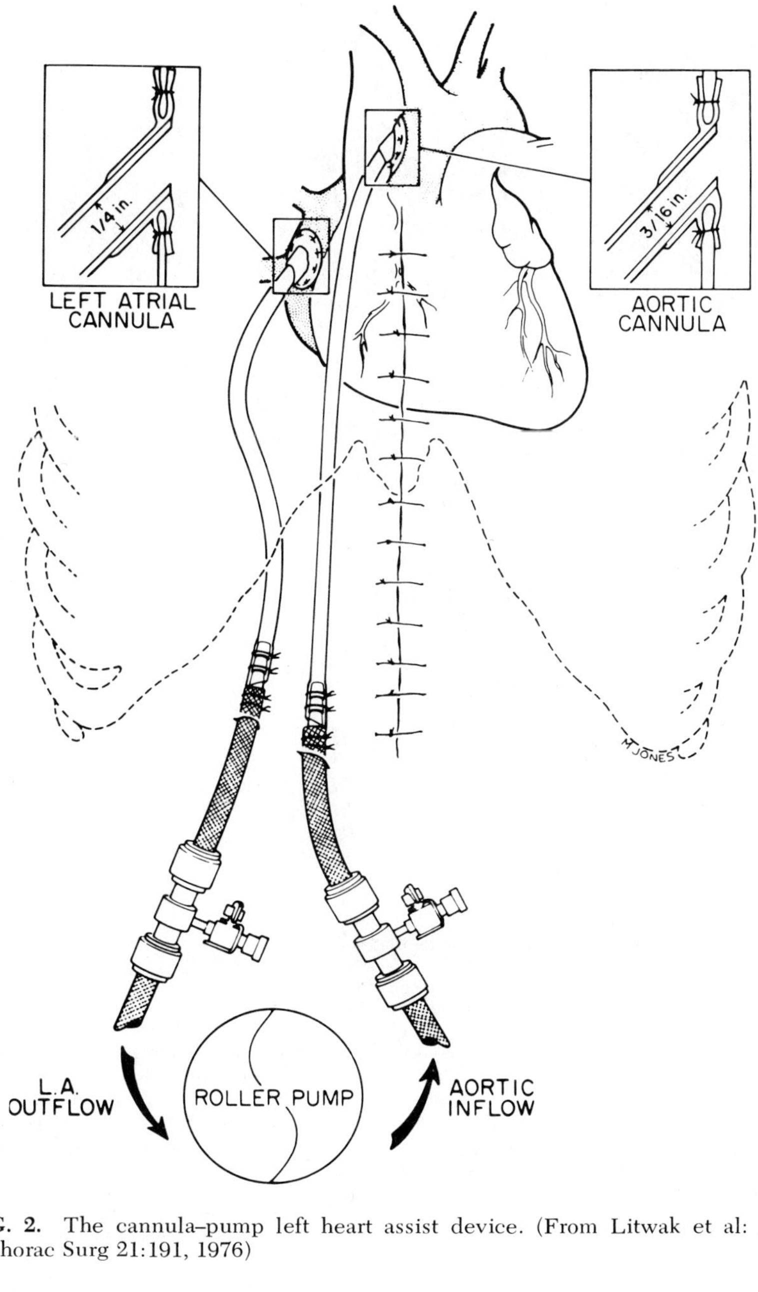

FIG. 2. The cannula–pump left heart assist device. (From Litwak et al: Ann Thorac Surg 21:191, 1976)

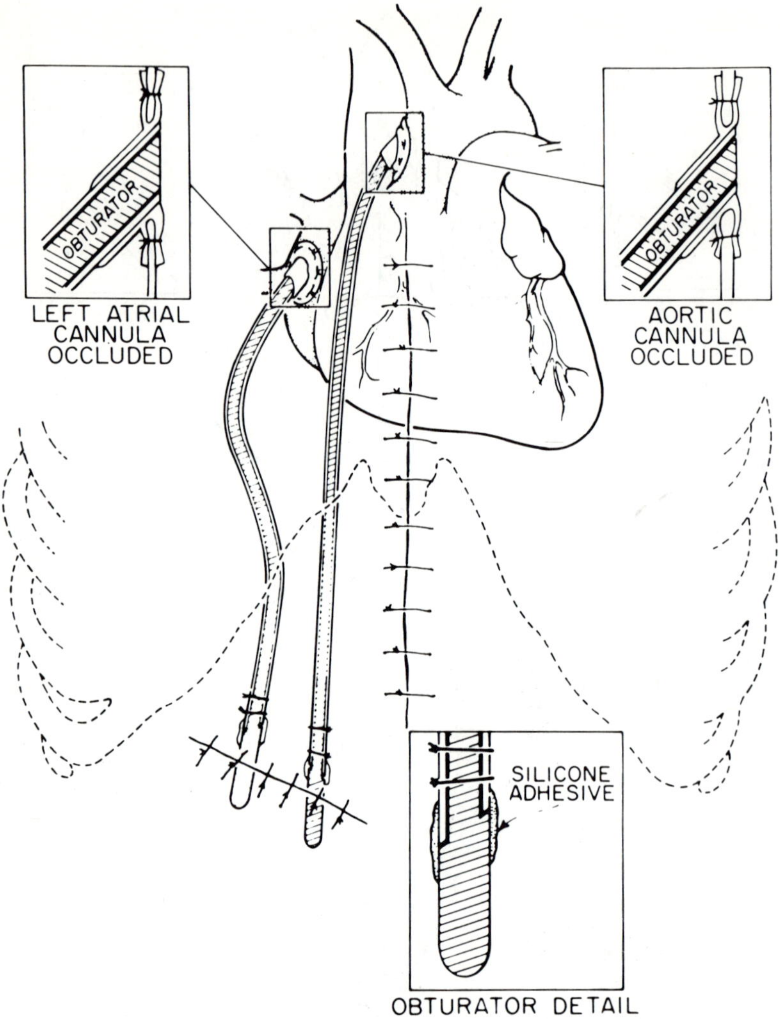

FIG. 3. Separation of the patient from the assist device is accomplished by exposing the distal cannula tips in their subcutaneous location through a small incision (bottom inset). The pump connections are separated from the cannulas, the obturators slipped into place and secured with ligatures and silicone elastomer glue. They are then left permanently in situ. (From Litwak et al: Ann Thorac Surg 21:191, 1976)

to minimize the potential of infection. Thus, the connections between the extracorporeal tubing loop and the LHAD cannulas are made in the subcutaneous plane of the right upper quadrant of the abdomen (Fig. 2).

In the operating room, LHAD flow rate is guided by LA and systemic arterial pressures. Once hemodynamic stability has been established and conventional cardiopulmonary bypass has been discontinued and decannulation carried out, partial heparin reversal is accomplished with protamine sulfate (1 mg/kg). This allows satisfactory hemostasis to be established while the LHAD continues to function at minimal levels of anticoagulation. Thereafter, the whole blood activated coagulation time[14] (ACT) is maintained between 110 and 140 seconds by hourly administration of small increments of heparin[15] (3 to 10 IU/kg). After closure of the sternum, the patient is moved to the intensive care unit (ICU) with the LHAD pump operating on battery power during the transfer.

In the ICU, a Swan-Ganz thermistor catheter is passed and TSBF measured by the thermodilution method. Knowledge of TSBF and LV filling pressures allows logical decisions to be made regarding LHAD flow rate and the possible need for blood volume augmentation. It is desirable to maintain TSBF at or above 2.5 liters/minute/meter^2 at mean LA pressures below 20 mm Hg.

Calculation of the percent LV contribution to TSBF is performed by using the formula:

$$\text{Percent LV contribution to TSBF} = \frac{\text{TSBF/minute} - \text{LHAD flow/minute}}{\text{TSBF/minute}} \times 100$$

As the LV contribution to TSBF increases (in the presence of acceptable levels of LA pressure), it is possible to slowly reduce the LHAD flow rate. With relatively low LHAD flows of 500 ml or less, it has been our practice to administer additional heparin (ACT level maintained between 160 to 200 seconds) to minimize thromboembolic potential due to blood velocity reduction through and increased residence time in the LHAD circuit. When it is determined that the LV is providing at least 90 percent of the TSBF (and TSBF remains at or above 2.5 liters/minute/meter^2 at satisfactory LV filling pressures), LHAD support is terminated.

Separation of the patient from the LHAD is readily accomplished by simply performing a small right subcostal incision using local infiltration anesthesia over the cannula-pump tubing junctions (Fig. 3). The pump is turned off, separation achieved, and the obturator of each cannula inserted, thereby obliterating the cannula lumen. Each obturator-cannula junction is secured with several heavy polyester ligatures and silicone glue and the skin closed over the now occluded cannulas (Fig. 3).

CLINICAL EXPERIENCE

Fifteen patients who could not be separated from conventional cardiopulmonary bypass because of persistent LV dysfunction (despite adjuvant supportive therapy including IABC whenever possible) underwent circulatory assistance with the LHAD. All patients were in New York class 4-4,[16] and 14 of the 15 had 3 or more of the following preoperative criteria of left ventricular dysfunction: (a) congestive heart failure refractory to therapy, (b) marked cardiomegaly, (c) diffuse impairment of LV contractility, (d) LV end-diastolic pressure greater than or equal to 20 mm Hg, and (e) cardiac index less than 2.5 liters/minute/meter^2.

Patients requiring LHAD support could be categorized in 3 groups (Table 2). The first group (9 patients) represented 17.6 per-

TABLE 2. Patient Categories and Results of Support with Left Heart Assist Device

PATIENT CATEGORY	NUMBER OF PATIENTS	SEPARATED FROM LHAD	IN-HOSPITAL DEATHS SUBSEQUENT TO LHAD SEPARATION	HOSPITAL SURVIVORS	LATE DEATHS
Patients previously denied operation	9	8	3	5	1
Patients with cardiogenic shock or cardiac arrest	4	1	0	1	1
Intraoperative myocardial infarction (aortic stenosis)	2	1	1	0	—
Totals	15	10	4	6	2

cent of a total of 51 patients with advanced cardiac dysfunction who were accepted for operation principally because of the availability of the LHAD. All had previously been considered by their cardiologists at this or another institution to have deteriorated to a point where operation could no longer be advised if only conventional perioperative supportive measures were to be employed, or they were considered operable only with extreme risk. The LHAD was used as a desperation measure in a second group of 4 patients who were either in established cardiogenic shock or cardiac arrest before intracardiac surgery. A third category in which LHAD use was unanticipated consisted of 2 patients who developed intraoperative myocardial infarctions after undergoing valve replacement for severe aortic stenosis.

LHAD support was employed from 2 hours to 21 days with maximal flow rates varying from 1500 to 4500 ml/minute. Immediate hemodynamic stability was achieved in 14 of 15 patients. Five patients remained LHAD dependent and all subsequently succumbed. In these, the LV contribution to TSBF consistently remained below 20 percent. Ten patients were successfully weaned from the LHAD. In this group, the LV had improved sufficiently to contribute at least 80 percent of TSBF by the third postoperative day, thereby permitting separation from the LHAD. Six patients were hospital survivors (LHAD support periods varied from 42 to 114 hours). Four patients remain well, the longest, 2.1 years postoperative. In 2 of the survivors, it had not been possible to deploy an intra-aortic balloon, presumably because of extensive aortoiliac atherosclerotic obstruction.

Discussion

Improved techniques of protection and support of the myocardium have allowed frequently successful operative intervention in patients with advanced cardiac dysfunction who, in earlier years, would have been considered to be inoperable. Thus, with increasing frequency, patients with markedly reduced cardiac performance are being submitted to surgery. In these individuals, even a modest intraoperative decrement of their already compromised myocardial pumping capacity obviously can be life threatening. Thus, the importance of having mechanical circulatory support systems immediately available is apparent.

Once a decision has been made to deploy a circulatory support system, two operational criteria become important: First, the system should be capable of being introduced with reasonable rapidity, for considerable time will have already been expended in attempting to wean the patient from conventional cardiopulmonary bypass. Secondly, the methods should not require subsequent reentry of the thorax or abdomen for device separation, since patients requiring postperfusion circulatory support are precisely those in whom another major surgical procedure could be hazardous. Both IABC and the LHAD satisfy these two criteria.

As indicated earlier, use of IABC is always attempted prior to considering LHAD deployment. Both methods can be used concurrently and, whenever feasible, IABC is continued for a period of time after LHAD separation so that weaning from all mechanical support is carried out in a deliberately gradual fashion.

In addition to augmenting TSBF with the LHAD, LV preload is significantly reduced. The resulting diminution in LV radius and wall tension should somewhat reduce myocardial oxygen consumption ($M\dot{V}O_2$) in accordance with the Laplace relationship. However, as suggested by animal investigations,[17–23] the magnitude of $M\dot{V}O_2$ reduction under clinical conditions of partial LV bypass with the LHAD is presumably only a modest one. In the experimental animal, nonpulsatile total LV bypass reduced $M\dot{V}O_2$ in the nontraumatized beating heart to approximately half the control level.[20] Lesser degrees of bypass were associated with smaller decrements of $M\dot{V}O_2$. At 50 percent partial LV bypass, there was an approximate 20 percent reduction in $M\dot{V}O_2$ with significant shortening of the LV end-diastolic fiber length.[20–23] The fact that two-thirds (10 of 15) of the patients having partial LV bypass with the LHAD could ultimately be separated from the device indicates that LV functional recovery can occur under physiologic conditions where $M\dot{V}O_2$ reduction would be expected to be only modest. The question arises as to whether the often expressed desideratum of maximal reduction of $M\dot{V}O_2$ is an essential goal in designing left heart support devices. As mentioned previously, most experimental studies have shown an inverse relationship between the percentage of left heart volume bypassed and $M\dot{V}O_2$. However, it is pertinent that Schenk and his colleagues[24] did not observe a fall in $M\dot{V}O_2$ in dogs during partial left heart bypass and found that it actually increased in some animals. More recently Wakabayashi and associates[25] extended these observations and found that $M\dot{V}O_2$ was markedly decreased in ischemically induced cardiogenic shock but gradually increased under conditions of left heart bypass. It seems apparent that additional studies are required to clarify our understanding of the directional changes of $M\dot{V}O_2$ in the bypassed normal and diseased heart.

Despite present limited knowledge of precisely *how* and *why* partial LV bypass allows the diseased and surgically traumatized heart to improve its performance, our results (Table 2) support the hypothesis that total LV bypass is not an absolute sine qua non for recovery of cardiac contractile function in man. Hence, no attempt is made to achieve maximal LV bypass with the LHAD. Rather, the LHAD is adjusted so that it supplements whatever volume is being ejected by the LV to permit establishment of metabolically stable conditions (TSBF greater than or equal to 2.5 liters/ minute/meter^2) at satisfactory LV filling pressures.

As presently designed (using a roller pump), the LHAD provides essentially nonpulsatile flow. The potential physiologic advantages of pulsatility are clearly apparent, and it is possible that the approach recently described by Bregman in chapter 2, may offer a relatively simple means of accomplishing this. We have not yet elected to employ a pulsatile pumping mode for two reasons. First, both cannula diameters would have to be enlarged, and this would increase the technical problems of insertion (particularly the ascending aortic cannula if aortic valve replacement and multiple coronary artery bypass grafting had been done). Secondly, pulsatile flow would require a more complex system with addition of a sac-like ventricle and possible valves. The present minimal heparin requirements would almost certainly have to be increased since there is as yet no thromboresistant surface that has been shown to reliably retain these qualities over a period of one month of pumping. The need for additional heparin might increase the chance of bleeding in fresh postoperative patients.

Our early clinical experience with the LHAD has been encouraging. LHAD deployment, operation, and patient separation have been relatively simple and uncomplicated. It is believed that the ability to carry out device separation from the patient without need for subsequent thoracic or abdominal reentry is a major asset of the method. The retained obturated cannulas have been well tolerated (the longest patient follow-up is now slightly over two years), an experience identical to that observed in dogs who have now been followed for four years. Although the LHAD will rarely be required, its capacity to augment TSBF while simultaneously reducing LV preload may be lifesaving in patients with severe postrepair pump failure.

SUMMARY

Patients with advanced cardiac dysfunction undergoing open intracardiac operation may require mechanical circulatory support to avoid the life-threatening consequences of low cardiac output if separation from conventional cardiopulmonary bypass (CPBP) cannot be accomplished. Fifteen patients in low cardiac output required support with a left heart assist device (LHAD) with flow from left atrium to ascending aorta. The LHAD was employed only after all other measures (including balloon pumping whenever possible) had failed to permit discontinuance of CPBP. Ten patients were ultimately separated from the LHAD, six were dismissed from the hospital, and four remain well (the longest, 2.1 years postoperative). It is believed that a major asset of the LHAD is that thoracic or abdominal reentry is not required when support is discontinued.

REFERENCES

1. Oldham HN Jr, Kong Y, Bartel AG, et al: Risk factors in coronary artery bypass surgery. Arch Surg 105:918, 1972
2. Lea RE, Tector AJ, Flema, RJ, et al: Prognostic significance of a reduced left ventricular ejection fraction in coronary artery surgery (abstract). Circulation 45, 46 (Suppl):II-49, 1972
3. Hammermeister KE, Kennedy JW: Predictors of surgical mortality in patients undergoing direct myocardial revascularization. Circulation 49, 50 (Suppl):II–112, 1974
4. Cohn PF, Gorlin R, Cohn LH, Collins JJ Jr: Left ventricular ejection fraction as a prognostic guide in surgical treatment of coronary and valvular heart disease. Am J Cardiol 34:136, 1974
5. Litwak RS, Silvay J, Gadboys HL, et al: Factors associated with operative risk in mitral valve replacement. Am J Cardiol 23:335, 1969
6. Appelbaum A, Kouchoukos NT, Blackstone EH, Kirklin JW: Early risks of open heart surgery for mitral valve disease. Am J Cardiol 37:201, 1976
7. Buckley MJ, Craver JM, Gold HK, et al: Intra-aortic balloon pump assist for cardiogenic shock after cardiopulmonary bypass. Circulation 47, 48 (Suppl):III-90, 1973
8. Berger RL, Saini VK, Ryan TJ, Sokol DM, Keefe JF: Intra-aortic balloon assist for postcardiotomy cardiogenic shock. J Thorac Cardiovasc Surg 66:906, 1973

9. Bregman D, Parodi EN, Malm JR: Left ventricular and unidirectional intra-aortic balloon pumping. J Thorac Cardiovasc Surg 68: 677, 1974
10. Parker FB Jr, Neville JF, Hanson EL, Webb WR: Intra-aortic balloon counterpulsation and cardiac surgery. Ann Thorac Surg 17:144, 1974
11. Litwak RS, Lajam F, Koffsky RM, et al: Obturated permanent left atrial and aortic cannulae for assisted circulation after cardiac surgery. Trans Amer Soc Artif Int Organs 19:243, 1973
12. Litwak RS, Koffsky RM, Lukban SB, et al: Implanted heart assist device after intracardiac surgery. New Engl J Med 291:1341, 1974
13. Litwak RS, Koffsky RM, Jurado RA, et al: Use of a left heart assist device after intracardiac surgery: Technique and clinical experience. Ann Thorac Surg 21:191, 1976
14. Hattersley PG: Activated coagulation time of whole blood. JAMA 196:150, 1966
15. Hill JD, Dontigny L, deLeval M, Mielke CH Jr: A simple method of heparin management during prolonged extracorporeal circulation. Ann Thorac Surg 17:129, 1974
16. New York Heart Association, Criteria Committee Nomenclature and Criteria for Diagnosis of Diseases of the Heart and Great Vessels, 7th ed. Boston, Little, Brown, 1973, p 286
17. Evans L, Matsuoka Y: The effect of various mechanical conditions on the gaseous metabolism and efficiency of the mammalian heart. J Physiol 49:378, 1915
18. Katz LN, Feinberg H: The relations of cardiac effort to myocardial oxygen consumption and coronary blood flow. Circ Res 6:656, 1958
19. Sarnoff SJ, Braunwald E, Welch GH Jr, et al: Hemodynamic determinants of oxygen consumption of the heart with special reference to the tension-time index. Am J Physiol 192:148, 1958
20. Dennis C, Hall DP, Morens JR, Senning Å: Reduction of the oxygen ultilization of the heart by left heart bypass. Circ Res 10:298, 1962
21. Baird RJ, LaBrosse CJ, Lajos TZ, Thomas GW: Effects of a selective bypass of the left ventricle. Circulation 27:835, 1963
22. Miller DR: Comparative effects of left atrial or left ventricular bypass on coronary sinus flow and oxygen usage in dogs. Ann Surg 179:830, 1974
23. Chiu C, Dennis C, Harris B: Response of myocardial fiber length to left heart bypass. J Surg Res 9:241, 1969
24. Schenk WG Jr, Delin NA, Camp FA, et al: Assisted circulation: An experimental evaluation of counterpulsation and left ventricular bypass. Arch Surg 88:327, 1964
25. Wakabayashi A, Kubo T, Gilman P, Zuber WF, Connolly JE: Oxygen consumption of the normal and failing heart during left heart bypass. J Thorac Cardiovasc Surg 70:9, 1975

CHAPTER 4

An Intracorporeal (Abdominal) Left Ventricular Assist Device, XXX: Clinical Readiness and Initial Trials in Man

John C. Norman

Supported in part by USPHS Contract NO1-HL-73-2946, The John & Mary R. Markle Foundation, The Kelsey & Leary Foundation, and The Mary A. Fraley Fund.

ABSTRACT

The purpose of this chapter is to present documenting evidence of the clinical readiness of an abdominal left ventricular assist device (ALVAD) according to NHLI criteria, and the initiation of clinical trials of this device in otherwise irretrievable adult postcardiotomy patients at the Texas Heart Institute of St. Luke's Episcopal and Texas Children's Hospitals. The ALVAD system has been developed, modified, and improved under NHLI auspices over the past eight years,† with annual reviews. Over 20,000 hours of in vivo testing in the calf have been accomplished in our laboratories. The current clinical trials underwent two federal reviews (May 22, 1973; and October 17, 1974) and were the topic of an ad hoc workshop at NHLI on October 28, 1973.‡ More recently, a consecutive series of 26 bovine ALVAD implantations were undertaken; acute and chronic hemodynamic effectiveness with maintenance or augmentation of the systemic circulation during profound ventricular unloading without undue blood trauma, intra- or extra-prosthetic thrombosis, or sepsis, was demonstrated; no biomaterials problems were encountered. In vivo reliability and durability, histologic and pathologic results were detailed and summarized and submitted to NHLI. Patient acceptability surveys and geometric and volumetric human configuration studies were analyzed. Categorizations of the patients at risk in our institutions and the needs for such a device were documented. The periods of intended use (two weeks to one month), weaning procedures, and the possibility of pump dependence have been discussed. The legal, moral, ethical, and informed consent issues were addressed and resolved. Clinical protocols (anesthesia, surgical, cardiologic, hematologic, engineering, computerized data acquisition, follow-up) and cost analyses were developed. The device has now been used in four terminal patients since December 1975; all subsequently succumbed, but their circulations were temporarily supported without biologic heart action for periods up to eight hours. Continued systematic, controlled clinical investigations of this nature are warranted. A current consent form is appended, and a comprehensive listing of pertinent references is included.*

**NIH Guide for Grants and Contracts, U.S. Dept. HEW 3:11, August 7, 1974.*
†In conjunction with Thermo Electron R&D Center, Waltham, Mass.
‡The Left Ventricular Assist Device: Assistance to the Failing Circulation, DHEW Publication No. (NIH) 75-626, U.S. Government Printing Office.

INTRODUCTION

The Cardiovascular Surgical Research Laboratories of the Texas Heart Institute of St. Luke's Episcopal and Texas Children's Hospitals in Houston were conceived of, designed, and built in 1971–72 with NHLI collaboration for the specific purposes of testing and evaluating left ventricular assist devices in the calf, with an ultimate goal of bringing these devices to orderly and systematic clinical trials in man. Over the past eight years, a goal-oriented approach involving planning, problem identification, and solving has evolved during a continued close collaboration with our engineering colleagues.

Our first proposal for ALVAD clinical trials (NO TE 2374-200), in response to RFP NHLI MADP-72-21 (Clinical Evaluation of Temporary Left Ventricular Assist Pumping) was submitted to NHLI on April 13, 1972. The trials were not subsequently approved. A second proposal for clinical trials was submitted on May 2, 1973 (NO TE 2436-200) and reviewed on May 22, 1973. Again, clinical trials were not approved. However, in recognition of their importance and imminence, a Workshop on Left Ventricular Assist Pumping was scheduled and convened at NHLI on October 28, 1973. The interested reader is referred to the Report on the Left Ventricular Assist Device (Assistance to the Failing Circulation), DHEW Publication No. (NIH) 75-626, prepared by NHLI staffers, Ruth J. Hegyeli, M.D. and Michael R. Machesko, B.A., January 11, 1974, wherein much of our data is summarized.

Our progress over the intervening year was reviewed at NHLI on October 17, 1974, and again on May 15, 1975, and clinical investigations began in our institutions in November 1975. The first clinical trial was undertaken on December 23, 1975.

BACKGROUND

The concept of circulatory assistance is not new. The need for such temporary support for weeks to months has been recognized for more than a decade, and still exists. The most common form of acute, iatrogenic, potentially reversible circulatory failure in man is that following cardiopulmonary bypass. If reliable means were available to support temporarily the circulation of such patients, the current low mortality associated with open heart surgery would be further decreased and, perhaps, the indications for high-risk patients broadened. For example, following otherwise uncomplicated procedures, it is common for patients to require reinstitution of cardiopulmonary bypass for brief periods to allow the biologic left ventricle to resume its pumping function to support the peripheral and central circulations. There is a correlation between the duration of the necessary period of resupport with the degree of acute left ventricular decompensation encountered. The limitations of prolonged bypass are hemolysis, protein denaturation, the appearance of hemorrhagic diatheses, and sepsis along vascular access perfusion lines. Cardiopulmonary bypass is a controlled form of shock and applicable for only short periods of time.

The techniques proposed for circulatory assistance have included aortic bypass pumping *(vide supra)*, intra-aortic balloon pumping, counterpulsation with an ectopic ventricle, external regional counterpulsation, synchronous airway pulsation, venovenous oxygenation, venoarterial oxygenation, mechanical synchronous sternal compression, and left atrial to systemic arterial pumping by various means for short periods of time. All have been utilized in man with varying degrees of success.

In comparison, our abdominal left ventricular assist device is a true intracorporeal blood pump. Unlike the intra-aortic balloon pump, which augments existing circulation, the ALVAD is capable of generating flow up to 10 liters per minute, independent of an intact EKG signal, and can be conceived of as an implantable partial artificial heart or life-support system. Such concepts and principles must be submitted to peer review in the current climate of the increasing involvement of medicine, technology, industry, and government, with society. Clearly, clinical use of this device involves not only the aforementioned sectors, but also impinges on moral, legal, and ethical interests.

It should be emphasized that, over the past four years, these implications have been given careful consideration. The National Heart, Blood Vessel, Lung and Blood Act of 1972 reaffirms the responsibility for research and development in this area; there is to be both research into and establishment of programs dealing with devices and instrumentation. The details can be found in Sections 413(A), items 3 and 4. Legislation is not specified.

DESCRIPTION OF THE ABDOMINAL LEFT VENTRICULAR ASSIST DEVICE SYSTEM

The abdominal left ventricular assist device system includes the following major subsystems: (a) the left ventricular assist device; (b) the clinical drive console, and (c) the pneumatic pump monitor.

Abdominal Left Ventricular Assist Device

The ALVAD (Fig. 1) is a single-chambered implantable blood pump actuated by an external pneumatic drive console. The pumping chamber is symmetric about a central axis. It weighs 470 g, measures 17 cm in length, and has a maximum diameter of 6.3 cm with a displacement of 300 ml. It consists of a polyurethane bladder that collapses in three segments or lobes when pneumatic pressure is applied to the space between the bladder and the titanium housing. Unidirectional flow is imparted by caged silicone rubber disc valves at the inflow and outflow orifices. The design stroke volume of the ALVAD is 100 ml; flow rates in excess of 10 liters per minute have been measured in vivo. Polyester fibers (0.001-inches in diameter and 0.010-inches in length) coat all blood-contacting surfaces except the valve discs and outflow graft.* These fibers provide a matrix on which a bioderived blood-compatible surface develops, ie, a neointima on a substrate of fibrin and erythrocytes.

A unique characteristic of the ALVAD is its anatomic placement (Fig. 2). The pump is designed for abdominal placement to facilitate implantation without pulmonary compromise and to permit subsequent removal without thoracotomy. Blood is received from the apex of the left ventricle through a semiflexible transdiaphragmatic inlet tube and ejected into the infrarenal abdominal aorta via a tightly woven low-porosity polyester graft. Serial acute and chronic experiments in dogs and calves have indicated that: (a) the ALVAD is hemodynamically effective and mechanically reliable; (b) the configuration is practical; and (c) no untoward perturbation of cardiac function is demonstrable when

**Meadox Medicals low porosity, 6 Raritan Road, Oakland, N.J. 07436.*

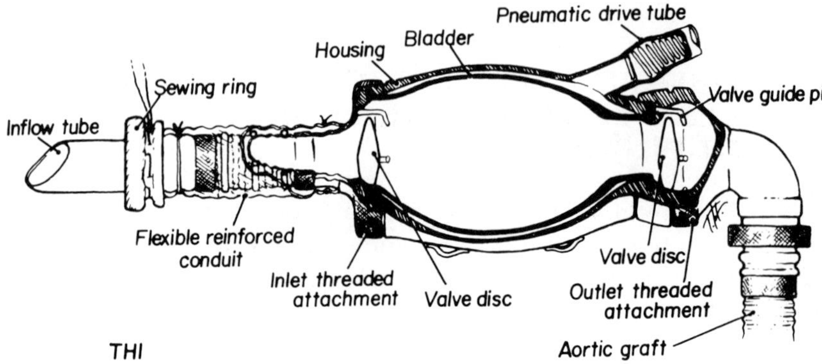

FIG. 1. The abdominal left ventricular assist device: cutaway illustration.

inflow tubes have been left in situ over extended periods (up to 289 days).

Another major prerequisite for clinical application of the ALVAD was the determination of its volumetric and geometric suitability relative to the anatomic variations and constraints in man. Human fitting studies included trial ALVAD fittings in 20 patients undergoing resections of abdominal aortic aneurysms and postmortem ALVAD implantations in 15 cadavers. No anatomic limitations were encountered in the trial fittings or cadaver implantations. Variations in left ventricular apex orientation were accommodated by adjustment of the flexible inlet tube. Variations in distance from the pump outlet to the abdominal aorta were accommodated by tailoring of the polyester outflow graft. In no instance was postmortem ALVAD implantation precluded by geometric or volumetric constraints.

Clinical Drive Console

For actuation and control of the ALVAD, it is necessary to have variable settings of pump chamber pressurization (0 to 400 mm Hg), vacuum-assisted pumping chamber filling (0 to 200 mm Hg), pulse duration (0 to 600 msec), and synchronized counterpulsation delay following QRS detection (100 to 1000 msec). To satisfy these requirements, an external clinical drive console has been designed and tested providing pneumatic drive and control, electronic logic, and failsafe mechanisms desirable for clinical

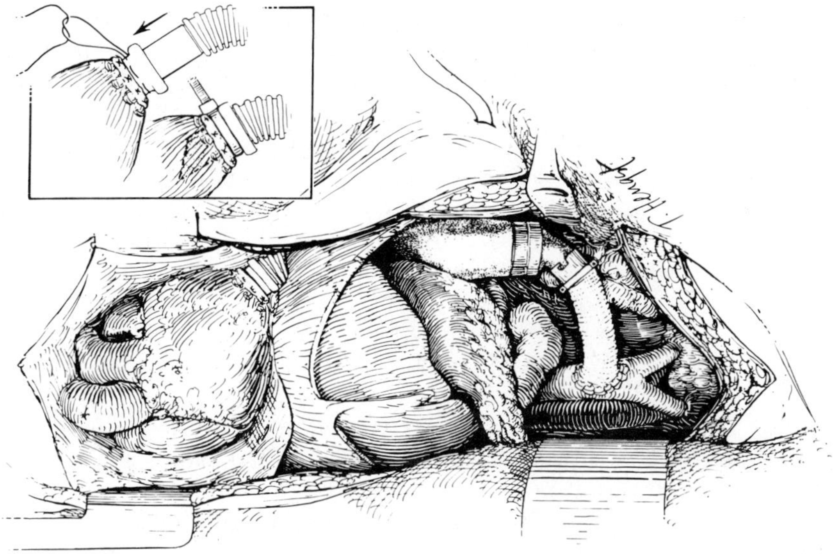

FIG. 2. Anatomic placement of the ALVAD (expanded).

use. There are two modes of operation: EKG-triggered synchronous counterpulsation, and variable fixed-rate asynchronous pumping. There are two pneumatic subsystems. The primary subsystem will operate in either mode; a secondary subsystem provides drive pressure at adjustable fixed rates, should the primary system fail for any reason. Both pneumatic subsystems allow adjustments of pump pressurization and pump ejection (systolic) time, with augmentation by vacuum-assisted filling available in the primary pumping module. Four failsafe functions are provided for (a) EKG interruption; (b) primary subsystem mechanical or electrical failure; (c) loss of external pneumatic power; and (d) loss of AC line power. The internal pneumatic and electrical power supplies permit fully portable operation of the console for periods of 50 minutes. A four-month console life test has been conducted in our laboratories without the occurrence of any failure that would cause discontinuation of pumping.

Pneumatic Pump Monitor

The pneumatic pump monitor (PPM) has been developed for control and quantitation of ALVAD function. This device consists of a pneumatic isolation piston and cylinder in the pump drive line, piston displacement transducer, drive-line pressure transducer, and an analogue computer with digital display and analogue outputs. By adjustment of the isolation piston displacement, the pump-stroke volume can be regulated to any percentage (20 to 95) of full capacity, thereby continuously avoiding pump bladder overcollapse with any possible denudation of developing neointima. The piston displacement and drive-line pressure transducer signals are utilized to compute pump stroke volume according to the formula:

$$SV = ApX - V_1 \left[P_T/(P_{atm} + P_T)\right]$$

where SV = stroke volume; Ap = piston area; X = piston displacement; V_1 = initial air volume within the isolation cylinder, drive line and pump housing; P_T = drive line pressure, and P_{atm} = atmospheric pressure. The computed stroke volume is multiplied by the pumping rate to yield pump minute flow. Digital data available from the PPM include (a) pump stroke volume (0 to 95 ml); (b) ALVAD beat rate (5 to 140 bpm), and (c) pump minute flow (0 to 13.3 liters per minute). In addition, drive line pressures (−200 to +400 mm Hg), rate of pump filling and ejection (0 to 1000 ml/sec), and duration of pump filling and ejection (0 to 600 msec) are available as analogue signals. Monitoring of these parameters allows maximum control, adjustment, and fine tuning of ALVAD assistance.

PATIENT SELECTION

Informed consent (Fig. 3) is obtained from all high-risk adult patients. Such patients, who cannot be weaned from cardiopulmonary bypass following conventional resuscitative measures, including intra-aortic balloon pumping (IABP), have constituted the first category of patients to be considered for ALVAD implantation.

A second category of patients are those who are not thought to be at high risk preoperatively, but who cannot be weaned from cardiopulmonary bypass with pharmacologic and IABP support. Informed consent is obtained from their nearest relatives.

A third category of patients as possible candidates are those

ST. LUKE'S EPISCOPAL HOSPITAL
Houston, Texas

Patient ________________________ **Hospital No.** _________________ **Date** _____

1. I understand that in a certain percentage of cardiovascular operative procedures, the natural heart is unable to resume adequate pumping to sustain life. I also understand that extensive laboratory and animal testing suggests that implantation of a temporary left ventricular assist pump in such cases may provide sufficient circulatory support to provide a rest period long enough to enable the natural heart to recover its pumping function.

2. I have asked Dr. __________________________________ to perform cardiovascular surgery on me in an attempt to correct my ____________________
____.

   (state name of problem to be surgically treated)

   If in the course of that surgery or the postoperative period, it is determined by Dr. __________________________________ that my natural heart is unable to resume adequate pumping to sustain my life, I hereby request and authorize him and whomever he may designate to proceed with use of an experimental temporary left ventricular assist device if in their judgment it can reasonably be expected to preserve my life.

3. I understand that the temporary left ventricular assist pumping device has been developed over the past eight years under the sponsorship of the National Heart and Lung Institute. I further understand that the device has been extensively tested in the laboratory and in animals, and has also been used in humans. I further understand that the positioning and nature of the device requires that, in addition to the surgery necessary for the procedure stated above, abdominal surgery will be required for implantation of the device, and, because it is temporary, a second operation under appropriate anesthesia will be necessary for its removal. I hereby consent to this second operation.

4. I understand the experimental temporary left ventricular assist pump will be utilized only after all other treatment alternatives have been exhausted, at which point it will be the only alternative which affords any possibility of preserving my life.

5. The potential complications associated with use of the device have been explained to me, and I understand that beyond the risks normally associated with any cardiovascular surgical procedure under general anesthesia, the most significant risks associated with use of the device are:

   a. Thromboembolism—the production of small clots which may become lodged in blood vessels and impair blood circulation to vital organs

   b. Impairment or loss of organ or body function

   c. Mechanical failure—the pump or one of its components might break down and fail to operate

   d. Pump dependence—the inability to discontinue assist pumping

6. I understand that if the device is used, I can anticipate essentially the same or more postoperative discomfort as that experienced by any patient following cardiovascular surgery. I understand that there may be additional or pro-

FIG. 3. Consent Form. (continues on next page)

longed discomfort due to a second abdominal operation for removal of the device. I also understand that use of the device would necessitate additional instrumentation and studies in order that adequate information can be obtained about mechanical function of the device. Such instrumentation and studies would consist of or be similar to those experienced in cardiac catheterization and the attendant discomfort would be essentially the same. I also understand that further studies, including cardiac catheterization, may be necessary following my discharge from the hospital.

7. I acknowledge that no guarantees have been made to me concerning the results of my surgery or the performance of the temporary left ventricular assist pump, should it be necessary to use it. However, I also understand that this temporary left ventricular assist system may not be available.

8. I understand that the operating surgeon will be occupied solely with the surgery and that the administration of the anesthetic(s) is an independent function. I hereby request and authorize Dr. Arthur Keats, or others he may deem advisable, to administer the anesthesia.

9. I hereby consent to the presence of nonmedical observers at my surgery and to the photographing of the operation to be performed, including appropriate portions of my body, to be used for medical, scientific and educational purposes as Dr. ______________________ or his designate may deem appropriate.

10. I hereby give my permission for St. Luke's Episcopal Hospital and the physicians providing my care to release any or all of the information contained in my medical records as in the judgment of Dr. ______________________ may be necessary to the proper scientific evaluation of the temporary left ventricular assist pump.

11. I understand that Dr. ______________________ and Dr. John C. Norman are available and willing to answer any questions I may have.

12. I understand I am free at any time to withdraw my consent to use of the assist device, recognizing that the exercise of such an option after the pump is in me would likely result in my death. It is understood that none of the foregoing is intended to release my physician, St. Luke's Episcopal Hospital, Texas Heart Institute, or their agents from liability for negligence.

____
Patient

WITNESSES:

______________________ **Witness**	______________________ **Address**
______________________ **Witness**	______________________ **Address**
______________________ **Witness**	______________________ **Address**
______________________ **Witness**	______________________ **Address**

FIG. 3. *(con't.)*

who have undergone open-heart procedures, have been weaned from cardiopulmonary bypass, but are unresponsive to increasing concentrations of vasopressors during intra-aortic balloon pumping in the recovery rooms. Informed consent is obtained from their relatives. In the first two categories, maximum efforts are exerted to reestablish ventricular function and to obtain adequate cardiac output using pharmacologic agents combined with partial cardiopulmonary bypass support and intra-aortic balloon pumping for a minimum of 30 to 60 minutes.[1,2] The decision to implant the ALVAD requires the agreement of the surgeon(s) and attending anesthesiologists or cardiologists that all acceptable and reasonable measures to restore cardiac function have been exhausted. This decision is reflected in the patient's record. Similar decisions are reached in the recovery rooms or intensive care units to return deteriorating patients to the operating rooms for ALVAD implantation.

INFORMED CONSENT

Informed consent is obtained from high-risk patients. In instances where informed consent cannot be obtained from the patient, it is obtained from the nearest relative. This consent (Fig. 3) form reflects serial legal consultations of Attorney Richard Bergner of the Texas Heart Institute Human Studies Committee, along with William J. Curran, Frances Lee Professor of Legal Medicine of the Harvard School of Public Health, and Attorney Henry C. Reinhard, Administrator of the Fort Worth Children's Hospital. It has been modified according to the recommendations of the NHLI Workshop on Left Ventricular Assist Pumping (DHEW Publication No. NIH 75-626, January 11, 1974) and those of the Human Studies Committee of the Texas Heart Institute and the Research and Publications Committee of the St. Luke's Episcopal and Texas Children's Hospitals. The informed consent statement contains the basic elements outlined in The Institutional Guide to DHEW Policy on Protection of Human Subjects (DHEW Publication No. NIH 72-102, December 1971). Conversations during the explanation of the consent form are tape recorded and submitted to federal auspices.

PATIENT MANAGEMENT

The patient management protocol for ALVAD implantation addresses the following specific areas:

1. Pump implantatation in the operating room
2. Patient transport to the recovery room (ALVAD suite)
3. Postoperative clinical management
4. Pumping modes
5. Patient weaning options
6. Pump removal
7. Pump dependence

Pump Implantation

ALVAD implantation can be performed in any of our eight cardiovascular surgical suites (Fig. 4). The basic techniques of anastomosis of the outflow graft to the infrarenal abdominal aorta, left ventricular apical excision, and inflow tube insertion developed in calves are utilized in man. The primary steps of clinical implantation are:

1. Continuation or reinstitution of total cardiopulmonary bypass
2. Reinsertion of a left ventricular sump via the right superior pulmonary vein–left atrial junction
3. Extension of the median sternotomy into the abdomen, to and around the umbilicus (Fig. 5)
4. Anastomosis of the outflow graft to the infrarenal abdominal aorta with care being taken to avoid the IABP pump cable, if present (Fig. 6a-b)
5. Suturing of the Teflon felt sewing ring to the left ventricular apex (to the left of the terminal radicals of the left anterior descending coronary artery) (Fig. 6c)
6. Fashioning of a small diaphragmatic incision
7. Cross-clamping of the ascending aorta proximal to the aortic perfusion cannula
8. Circular excision of the left ventricular apex within the Teflon felt sewing ring (Fig. 6d)
9. Continuation of left ventricular drainage

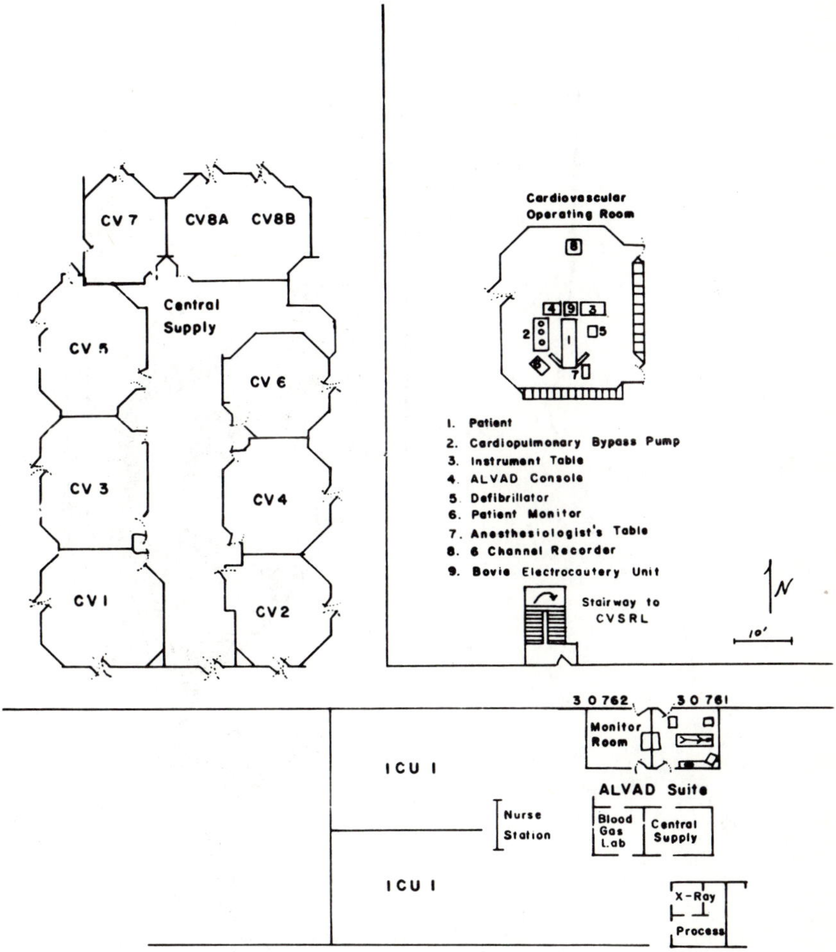

FIG. 4. Floor plan of Texas Heart Institute Cardiovascular Surgical Facilities with representative details of equipment in each operating room and the location of the ALVAD suite. Intensive Care Units (ICU) 1, 2, 3, and 4 have a total of 100 beds.

10. Visual and digital examination of the left ventricular apical aperture
11. Connection of the ALVAD pumping chamber with its attached inflow tube to the outflow graft
12. Priming of the inflow tube, pump, and outflow graft with dextran
13. Insertion of the ALVAD inflow tube through the dia-

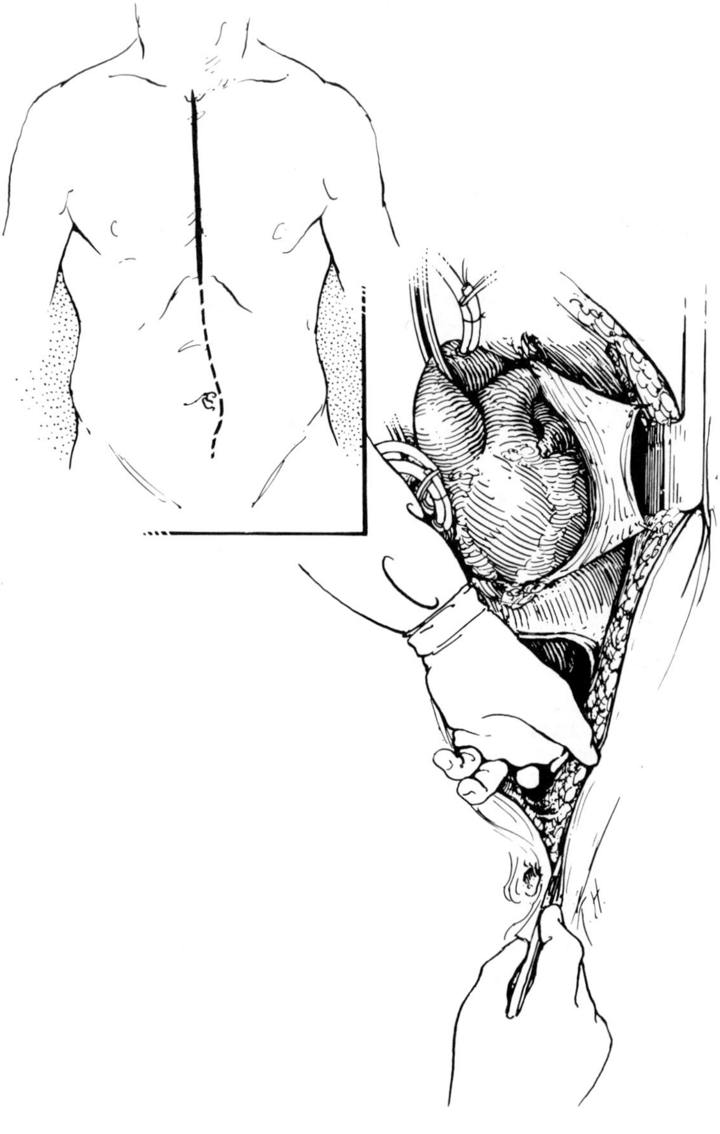

FIG. 5. ALVAD implantation: extension of median sternotomy into abdomen, to and around umbilicus.

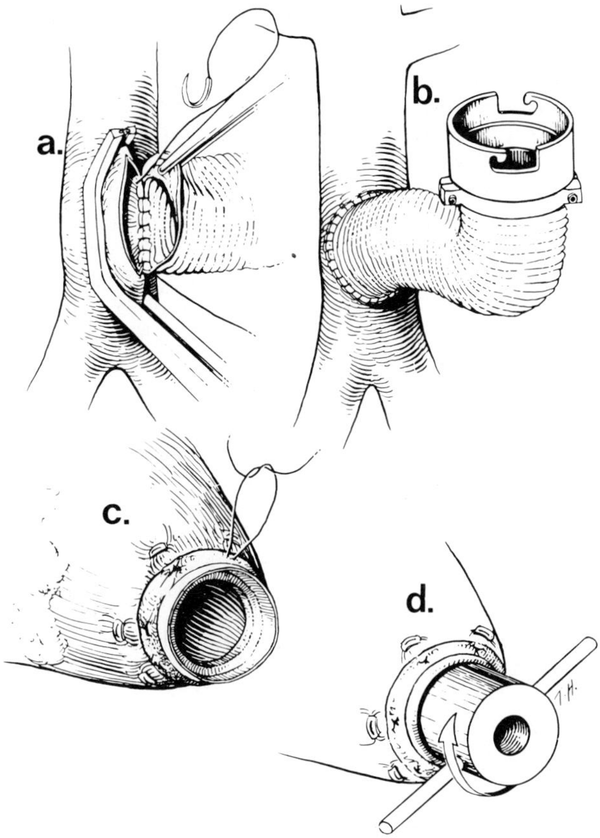

FIG. 6a and b. Anastomosis of the ALVAD outflow graft to the infrarenal aorta; **c.** Teflon felt sewing ring sutured to left ventricular apex; **d.** circulator excision of left ventricular apex within Teflon felt sewing ring.

phragmatic incision and apical aperture into the left ventricular apex

14. Exteriorization of the ALVAD pneumatic drive line through a small left flank incision in the midsuprailiac line
15. Evacuation of air from the ascending aorta proximal to the perfusion cannula
16. Evacuation of air from the ALVAD outflow graft
17. Removal of cross-clamps from the ascending aorta and ALVAD outflow graft
18. Pumping of a single ALVAD stroke to allow evacuation of air from the outflow graft

19. Reevacuation of any residual air from the ascending aorta
20. Initiation of ALVAD asynchronous pumping at low rates (35 to 45 bpm)
21. Initiation of weaning from cardiopulmonary bypass
22. Removal of the left ventricular sump from the right superior pulmonary vein–left atrial juncture
23. Placement of an overlapping circumferential purse-string suture around the sump aperture
24. Insertion of the left ventricular pressure transducer-tipped catheter through this purse-string suture and exteriorization of the transducer catheter and the purse-string suture through a 15-cm/3-mm Teflon tube via the right second intercostal space
25. Insertion of left ventricular epicardial bipolar pacemaking wires
26. Closure

ALVAD Pumping Modes

The clinical drive console can be adjusted to obtain any of the following pumping modes:

1. Low-rate asynchronous (35 to 45 bpm)
2. Asynchronous (45 to 140 bpm)
3. Synchronous counterpulsation (20 to 140 bpm)
4. Intermittent synchronous counterpulsation (1:1, 1:2, . . . , 1:10)

LOW-RATE ASYNCHRONOUS PUMPING. This pumping mode (35 to 45 bpm) is achieved by pumping at a low fixed-beat rate. The advantages of low-rate asynchronous pumping are simplicity of operation, and obviation of the necessity for a stable EKG. Low-rate asynchronous pumping is used for the initiation of ALVAD assistance. Initial start-up and increasing level of assistance is greatly simplified. Low-rate asynchronous pumping is also indicated in the recovery phase when only partial assistance is required.

ASYNCHRONOUS PUMPING. This pumping mode (45 to 140 bpm) has been utilized routinely for chronic ALVAD experiments in calves and during certain periods of our first four clinical investigations. The advantages of asynchronous pumping are that a stable EKG is not required, and the evaluation of left ventricular performance during weaning may be obtained by monitoring the aortic pressure for evidence of cardiac ejection in the absence of a left ventricular pressure trace.

SYNCHRONOUS COUNTERPULSATION. This pumping mode is achieved using the processed EKG synchronization signal. The ALVAD is therefore synchronized with the left ventricular beat rate and stroke volume. Otherwise stated, the ALVAD fills during left ventricular systole and ejects during ventricular diastole (counterpulsation). The advantages of the synchronous pumping are consistent and continuous EKG-triggered left ventricular assistance (reduced LV work, minimal myocardial energy consumption, and increased diastolic systemic perfusion), and the correspondence of ALVAD filling period with left ventricular systole utilizing filling left ventricular ejection.

INTERMITTENT SYNCHRONOUS COUNTERPULSATION. This pumping mode is achieved electronically by selecting one of the following ALVAD ejection/R-R interval ratios—1:1, 1:2, . . . , 1:10. Intermittent synchronous counterpulsation is indicated in the recovery phase when partial assistance is required during synchronous pumping.

Patient-Weaning Options

If there is a return of left ventricular function, three weaning options are available for discontinuation of ALVAD assistance:

1. Reduced ALVAD filling vacuum during synchronous counterpulsation
2. Intermittent synchronous counterpulsation
3. Progressively lower rate asynchronous pumping

The clinical drive console can be adjusted to provide any of these weaning options.

REDUCED ALVAD FILLING VACUUM DURING SYNCHRONOUS COUNTERPULSATION. This weaning option can be achieved by decreasing the regulated ALVAD filling vacuum. As the filling vacuum is reduced, ALVAD filling (ventricular ejection) impedance is increased. The left ventricle must therefore develop a greater pressure to achieve the same stroke volume. The level of vacuum is variable between 0 and −200 mm Hg and is monitored during weaning.

INTERMITTENT SYNCHRONOUS COUNTERPULSATION. This weaning option is achieved electronically by selecting one of the following ALVAD ejection/R-R interval ratios—1:1, 1:2, . . . , 1:10. This weaning mode can also be used in conjunction with a reduced ALVAD filling vacuum. This weaning option allows pump rates as low as 5 to 20 bpm at an assist ratio of 1:10.

PROGRESSIVELY LOWER RATE ASYNCHRONOUS PUMPING. This weaning option is achieved by decreasing the asynchronous pumping rate in increments of 5 bpm to a minimum rate of 35 to 45 bpm. This weaning option can also be used in conjunction with a reduced ALVAD filling vacuum.

ALVAD Removal

Following implantation, ventricular recovery, and weaning procedures, pump removal is necessary. The ALVAD can be removed through the original abdominal incision. The inflow tube can be detached from the pump body, oversewn, and left in situ. The outflow graft can similarly be divided and oversewn. Previous bovine experiments have demonstrated that retained ALVAD inflow tubes cause no significant left ventricular dysfunction.

Pump Dependence

One of the major thrusts of our initial clinical studies is to determine whether or not temporary left ventricular assistance allows intrinsic left ventricular reparative processes to occur. In spite of our best efforts to select, support, and wean ALVAD recipients, some may become pump dependent. In our current end-stage patient population this has occurred in each instance.

In the case of pump dependence, the situation presents the physicians and families with the same problems as termination of unsuccessful intra-aortic balloon pumping or cardiopulmonary bypass.

LOGISTICS

Initial System Set-up and Check-out

When our Circulatory Support Service is notified that a candidate for ALVAD implantation has been identified, the clinical drive console, pneumatic pump monitor, and a six-channel chart recorder are transferred from the ALVAD monitoring suite in the recovery rooms to the operating room involved, by the engineering members of the group. During ALVAD implantation, the clinical drive console system functions are checked for proper operation. When not in use, the console is further checked each week according to the following protocol:

1. The console is connected to external AC power, air, and vacuum outlets.
2. The ALVAD drive line is connected to a simulated load, consisting of a transparent ALVAD housing, pump bladder, capped inlet, and outlet with variable resistance.
3. The console internal CO_2 supply is turned on and the tank gauge pressure observed for proper indication of 900 psi.
4. Proper function of the console AC power supply (Elgard Model UPS 501 uninterruptible AC power source) is verified as follows:
   a. The main AC power switch-circuit breaker is set to the ON position. The front panel indicators are observed to determine that the AC POWER ON lamp lights and remains on, and the REVERSE TRANSFER lamp lights.
   b. The battery switch-circuit breaker is set to the ON position, and the REVERSE TRANSFER lamp is observed to determine that it goes off. The OUTPUT VOLTAGE meter is observed to indicate 117.5 VAC.
   c. The AC power is momentarily disconnected, and the OUTPUT VOLTAGE meter is observed to continue to indicate 117.5 VAC without interruption in any fashion. The AC OFF and REVERSE TRANSFER lamps are observed to remain on and off, respectively. The BATTERY VOLTAGE meter is observed to indicate a fully charged condition of 84 VDC. The BATTERY LOW lamp is observed to remain off. This lamp only lights when approximately 3 minutes of battery power remain.
   d. External AC power is reapplied, and the AC OFF and AC ON lamps are observed for proper indication.
5. The console malfunction warning lights are tested as follows:
   a. The EKG-FIXED RATE mode switch is placed in the EKG position.
   b. The warning light NORMAL-TEST switch is placed in

the TEST position, and the six warning lights (EKG INTERRUPT, HEART RATE HIGH, HEART RATE LOW, PRIMARY SYSTEM FAILURE, EXTERNAL AIR SUPPLY FAILURE, and EXTERNAL AC POWER FAILURE) are observed to light.

6. The patient EKG and aortic pressure signals cable from the OR monitor and are connected to high-level input connectors on the clinical console, and are displayed on the integral four-channel oscilloscope.
7. Proper function of the pneumatic system is verified as follows:
   a. The PNEUMATIC SUPPLY PRESSURE gauge is observed to indicate 30 psi when the external air supply line is connected.
   b. The external air supply is momentarily disconnected and the PNEUMATIC SUPPLY PRESSURE gauge is observed to continue to indicate 30 psi from the internal CO_2 supply. In addition, the FAILURE OF EXTERNAL AIR SUPPLY lamp is observed to light.
   c. The external air supply is restored and the FAILURE OF EXTERNAL AIR SUPPLY lamp is observed to go off.
   d. The primary unit pressure and vacuum regulators are checked by rotating the regulator control knobs in a clockwise direction and observing the PRIMARY UNIT DRIVE PRESSURE and PRIMARY UNIT VACUUM gauges for increasing levels of pressure and vacuum. The regulator control knobs are rotated counterclockwise, and the gauges are observed for decreasing levels of pressure and vacuum. The secondary unit drive pressure is checked similarly.
8. The primary system electronics and pneumatics are checked as follows:
   a. The EKG–FIXED RATE mode selector switch is placed in the FIXED RATE position and the FIXED RATE lamp is observed to light.
   b. The PRIMARY SYSTEM RATE control is adjusted to 85 bpm.
   c. The PRIMARY SYSTEM EJECTION DURATION control is adjusted to 175 msec.
   d. The PRIMARY SYSTEM DRIVE and VACUUM PRESSURES are adjusted to 6 psi and 50 inches, H_2O, respectively.
   e. The primary unit is then activated, and proper function is verified by observation of the simulated load and PPM digital display, ie, stroke volume = 85 ml, beat rate = 85 bpm, flow = 7.2 liters/minute.
   f. The EKG INPUT LEVEL selector switch is placed in the HIGH LEVEL position.

g. The EKG TRIGGERING MODE selector switch is placed in the FIXED, QR, and RS position, and the QRS detection lamp is observed to light with each detected QRS complex.
h. The EKG–FIXED RATE mode selector switch is placed in the EKG position, and the EKG lamp is observed to light.
i. The primary unit is then activated and proper function is verified by observation of the simulated load and PPM digital display, ie, stroke volume = 85 ml, beat rate = patient's rate, and flow = 85 ml × patient's rate in bpm.
j. Proper function of the HEART RATE HIGH-HEART RATE LOW controls are verified as follows.
   (1) The HEART RATE HIGH LIMIT control is adjusted to less than or equal to the patient's rate.
   (2) The HEART RATE HIGH warning lamp is observed to light.
   (3) The primary system is observed to switch automatically to fixed-rate operation, lighting the FIXED RATE lamp.
   (4) The HEART RATE HIGH LIMIT control is adjusted to exceed the patient's rate.
   (5) The EKG FAILURE, RESET switch is depressed, and the primary system is observed to resume operation in the EKG mode, lighting the EKG lamp and turning off the HEART RATE HIGH lamp.
   (6) The HEART RATE LOW LIMIT control is adjusted to greater than or equal to the patient's rate.
   (7) The HEART RATE LOW warning lamp is observed to light.
   (8) The primary system is observed to switch automatically to fixed rate operation, lighting the FIXED RATE lamp.
   (9) The HEART RATE LOW LIMIT control is adjusted to less than the patient's rate.
   (10) The EKG FAILURE RESET switch is depressed, and the primary system is observed to resume operation in the EKG mode, lighting the EKG lamp and turning off the HEART RATE LOW lamp.

9. The secondary system electronics and pneumatics are checked as follows:
   a. The SECONDARY SYSTEM RATE control is adjusted to 85 bpm.
   b. The SECONDARY SYSTEM EJECTION DURATION control is adjusted to 175 msec or 25 percent of the beat-to-beat interval.

c. The SECONDARY SYSTEM DRIVE PRESSURE is adjusted to 6 psig.
d. The secondary system is then activated by depressing the SECONDARY SYSTEM TEST switch, and proper function is verified by observation of the dummy load and PPM digital display, ie, stroke volume = 85 ml, beat rate = 85 bpm, and flow = 7.2 liters/minute.

10. The PRIMARY SYSTEM FAILSAFE mechanism is tested as follows.
    a. While the primary system is operating, the HIGH PRESSURE LIMIT is adjusted to less than or equal to the indicated mean drive line pressure.
    b. The console is observed to switch automatically to secondary system operation, lighting the PRIMARY SYSTEM FAILURE lamp.
    c. The FAILSAFE HIGH PRESSURE LIMIT is adjusted to exceed the indicated mean drive line pressure by 20 mm Hg.
    d. The FAILSAFE, RESET switch is depressed, and the primary system is observed to resume operation.
    e. The FAILSAFE LOW PRESSURE LIMIT is adjusted to greater than or equal to the indicated mean drive line pressure.
    f. The console is observed to switch automatically to secondary system operation, lighting the PRIMARY SYSTEM FAILURE lamp.
    g. The FAILSAFE LOW PRESSURE LIMIT is adjusted to 20 mm Hg less than the indicated mean drive line pressure.
    h. The FAILSAFE, RESET switch is depressed, and the primary system is observed to resume operation.

This completes the ALVAD system set-up and check-out. During the weekly check-out procedures when the clinical drive console is not in use, an EKG simulator is used to supply a test electrocardiographic signal.

Clinical Drive Console Operation

Following ALVAD implantation, left ventricular assistance is initiated in the asynchronous mode at low rates (35 to 45 bpm). As cardiopulmonary bypass is decreased, the asynchronous pumping rate is gradually increased in increments of 5 bpm until the pump rate equals the patient's heart rate; then synchronous pumping is initiated. During this time, blood volume is restored, acid-base balance is corrected as necessary, and hemostasis is achieved. During initial and early left ventricular assistance, the drive console controls are always adjusted to maximize the pump stroke volume (ie, a stroke volume without pump bladder overcollapse)* and minute flow and to achieve minimal left ventricular pressure. The pumping capacity of the ALVAD is fill limited rather than ejection limited because sufficient power is available to eject whatever blood is received in the pumping chamber. The filling rate is thus the primary determinant of stroke volume, which may be influenced by manual adjustment of the drive console controls. During synchronous counterpulsation, reiterative adjustment of ejection duration, ejection delay after QRS detection, and vacuum-assisted filling pressure allow maximization of pump filling rate and consequently, pump diastolic volume. Maximum stroke volume is achieved by adjustment of drive pressure to overcome pump ejection impedance.

Observation of the pneumatic pump monitor digital and analogue data during drive console adjustment allows maximal control and "fine tuning" of ALVAD assistance. For example, to achieve a maximum ALVAD minute flow of 6.6 liters per minute during synchronous pumping at 85 bpm and a mean aortic pressure of 110 mm Hg, the following drive console adjustments are made: ejection duration, 175 msec; ejection delay, 350 msec after QRS detection; pump drive and filling pressures, 250 and −100 mm Hg, respectively. These drive console settings will result in a pump filling duration of 400 msec, peak filling and ejection rates of 600 and 800 ml/sec, respectively, and a stroke volume of 78 ml.

The patient is monitored for a stabilization period of one to three hours in the operating room. When the patient is judged to be ready for transfer to the ALVAD monitoring suite, the EKG leads and aortic and left ventricular pressure transducers, are transferred to the clinical console for monitoring during transport, and the console is converted to operation on internal electrical and pneumatic power sources. After arrival in the intensive care

**Pump bladder overcollapse results in contact between opposing internal bladder surfaces with increased blood trauma and possible denudation of developing neointima. Overcollapse of the ALVAD pump bladder occurs at stroke volumes greater than 95 ml. The pump stroke volume is always limited to less than 95 ml to avoid this problem. Conventional pharmacologic and mechanical methods of circulatory support can be used in conjunction with the ALVAD. Cardiopulmonary bypass can be continued and weaned; IABP actuation should be discontinued.*

unit, the clinical drive console is returned to operation on external AC power, air, and vacuum.

Maximum synchronous left ventricular assistance (ie, maximum ALVAD stroke volume, maximum minute flow, and minimum left ventricular pressure) is continued throughout the first day after ALVAD implantation. The level of left ventricular assistance is dictated by the patient's clinical condition. During the postimplantation period, left ventricular (LV) function during less than maximum synchronous ALVAD assistance is evaluated. This reduction in left ventricular unloading is accomplished by decreasing vacuum-assisted pump filling pressure or slight changes in ejection delay to cause a reduction in pump filling rate and stroke volume as indicated by the pneumatic pump monitor. If the patient remains stable, ALVAD support can be continued at reduced levels of left ventricular assistance. If the patient does not remain stable, maximum left ventricular assistance is reinstituted. If the patient remains stable with partial support for at least 48 hours, initiation of weaning from left ventricular assistance can be attempted. Similar procedures for patient weaning from intraaortic balloon pump assistance have been developed and implemented during the past 36 months by our clinical studies group. Initiation of weaning is accomplished by pumping asynchronously at a rate equal to the patient's heart rate. The drive console ejection duration, drive, and vacuum-assisted filling pressure controls will be adjusted to achieve stroke volumes between 30 and 70 ml. If the patient's condition remains stable, this mode of left ventricular support will be continued for 24 to 48 hours. The patient's status can be quantitated by comparisons of current and computer-stored data. Left ventricular function studies are performed during synchronous and asynchronous pumping at various levels of left ventricular support, and with the pump turned off for brief periods. The results of these studies determine the mode of pumping to be used during continued weaning. Either asynchronous pumping at rates less than the patient's heart rate or semisynchronous pumping (1:2, 1:3, 1:4, . . . , etc, LV assist: R-R interval) can be chosen to provide the level of support required by the patient. These left ventricular function studies will be repeated each following day, and the level of support will be gradually reduced as indicated by the patient's condition. It is anticipated that sufficient recovery of left ventricular function to allow pump removal will have occurred by 14 days or earlier, and left ventricular support at this time will be minimal. If this is the case, the patient will be returned to the operating room and the pump will be removed. It is, of course, difficult to predict the period of left ventricular assistance which any patient will require; some may recover earlier than 14 days, and some may require continued support and will be considered pump dependent.

INSTRUMENTATION

In any of our eight open-heart operating rooms, the available instrumentation consists of the fixed overhead Statham operating room monitors (EKG, EEG, and arterial pressure), the ALVAD clinical console with pneumatic pump monitor, and a six-channel chart recorder (Fig. 7). Initial EKG and aortic pressure signals are recorded from the OR monitor. These two data channels are recorded within minutes of patient selection. While the ALVAD is being implanted, the LV pressure transducer and pneumatic pump monitor are calibrated on the chart recorder. Channel 3 is the LV transducer output, while channels 4 through 6 are pump monitor signals (ie, stroke volume, minute output, and driveline pressure).

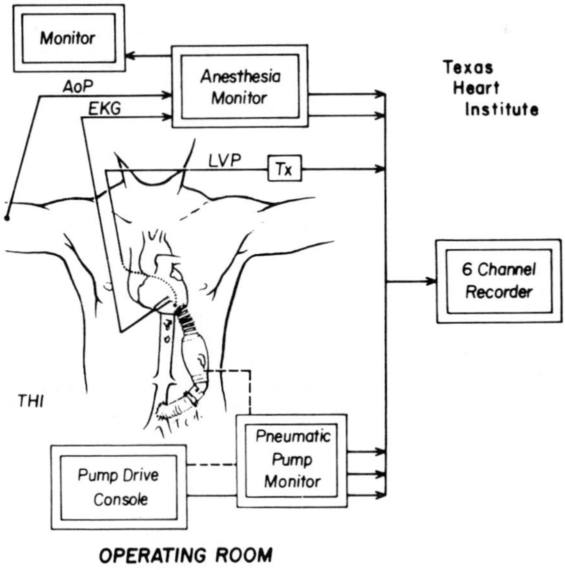

FIG. 7. Block diagram of THI operating room(s) ALVAD patient-monitoring instrumentation.

In the operating room, adjustments and studies have been undertaken in the following sequence, ie:

1. Initial asynchronous rates to assure pump filling
2. Systemic perfusion and maintenance of arterial pressure
3. Degree of LV unloading
4. Ability to synchronize with the biologic heart
5. Effects of synchronous counterpulsation timing on LV unloading and pump output

The operating room monitors display aortic pressure (AoP) and EKG, while the ALVAD clinical console's four-channel scope displays either AoP, LVP, or EKG, and the three pump monitor signals. Console adjustments are normally made based on AoP and stroke volume during asynchronous pumping. When synchronous pumping is begun, either the LV or EKG signals are displayed on the console's scope for pump delay timing adjustments.

If the circulatory status stabilizes, and the patient is judged ready for transport, the clinical console is connected to internal battery power. The console monitors EKG, AoP, LVP, and pump stroke volume while the patient and console are moved to the adjacent intensive care unit (ICU).

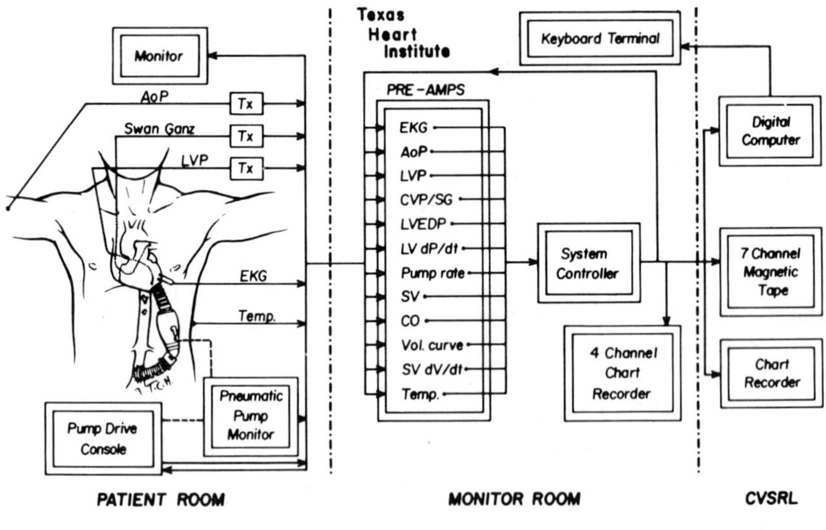

FIG. 8. Block diagram of intensive care unit (ALVAD suite)–Cardiovascular Surgical Research Laboratories data acquisition system.

ALVAD Suite Instrumentation

The patient arrives in the ICU supported by the ALVAD with the portable clinical console monitoring EKG, AoP, LVP, and pump stroke volume. The console is converted back to AC power and connected to the ALVAD suite instrumentation cable. The ALVAD suite instrumentation system is block diagrammed in Figures 8 and 9. As soon as the console is connected, the patient's nonfade room monitor displays the EKG, Ao, and LV pressures. Pump monitor outputs, patient data processing, and display are then controlled from a monitoring room which is separated from the ALVAD suite by a glass partition.

The amplifier system in the ALVAD monitoring room has 12 channels for signal processing. Channel 1 is an EKG amplifier; channels 2 through 4 are carrier-type pressure amplifiers for Ao, LV, and either PA or CV pressures. Channel 5 is a derivative computer (dP/dt) for LV pressure, and channel 6 is an amplifier of LVP for end-diastolic pressure (0 to 40 mm Hg). When the ALVAD clinical console is connected to the instrumentation system, channels 7 through 10 process pump monitor signals (ie, pump rate, stroke volume, minute output, and flow curve). Channel 11 is a derivative computer (dV/dt) of the flow curve (channel 10) to provide rate of flow for both filling and ejecting peak velocities. Channel 12 is a DC amplifier for the patient's temperature.

A system controller is connected to the amplifier system's output. The system controller routes the 12 data channels to display and storage devices. With this controller, any of the above signals can be displayed on the patient's monitor, and a four-channel chart recorder in the monitoring room. The clinical console still displays the driveline pressure, but can select any of the other signals (eg, LVP, SV, dV/dt) for its three remaining channels. This monitor is used in adjusting ALVAD pump control.

Physiologic data is displayed on the patient's monitor (ie, EKG, Ao, LV pressures, and either dP/dt, PA, or CV pressures). The four-channel chart recorder produces a permanent hard-copy record of pumping data (ie, stroke volume, minute output, flow rate, and LV pressure); any four channels can be recorded for permanent hard-copy comparisons.

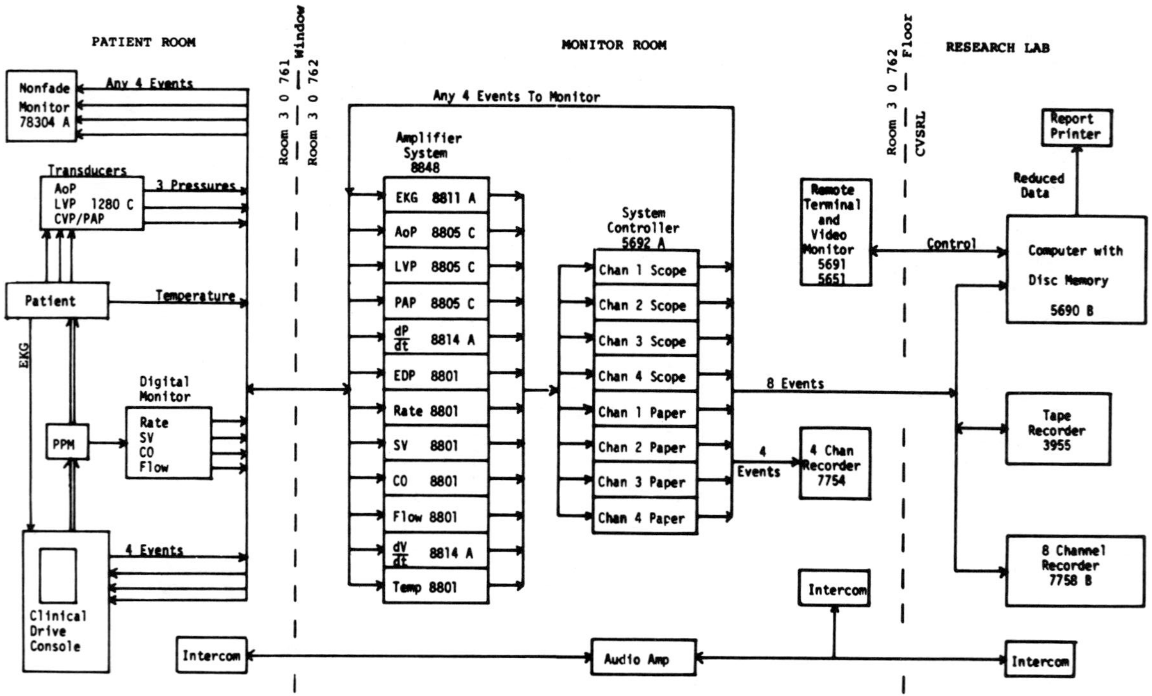

FIG. 9. Detailed block diagram of intensive care unit (ALVAD suite)—Cardiovascular Surgical Research Laboratories data acquisition system.

Remote Data Management and Processing

The Cardiovascular Surgical Research Laboratories (CVS-RL) are located on the floor directly above the clinical ALVAD monitoring suite. The preclinical studies on the ALVAD have been performed in the laboratories, and an advanced data management system is used for research procedures. The CVSRL data system is connected to the system controller in the clinical ALVAD monitoring suite. In the laboratories, a seven-channel FM tape recorder and an eight-channel chart recorder are calibrated and operated by the system controller on the floor below. This allows both on-line and off-line studies to be performed with any eight of the twelve monitoring channels without disturbing the clinical procedures.

A digital computer is used in the laboratories for experimental cardiac catheterization studies. A remote terminal and video display are located in the clinical ALVAD monitoring suite. The computer samples EKG, pressure, and thermodilution-type cardiac output data directly from the system controller by terminal command. The computer's 8K active memory processes simultaneous pressure data and displays both sampled analog waveforms and digital analyses on the video monitor (Fig. 10). The analyzed data is also stored on a 2.5 megabyte disc for later recall as requested from the terminal. A report of the data is printed (on request) by the computer for a permanent detailed record of all ALVAD patient courses during computer monitoring.

The computer can sample hemodynamic data both during and in the absence of ALVAD pumping. Typical sample data includes Ao, LV, and PA pressures simultaneously. The computer determines:

1. Ao systolic, diastolic, and mean pressure
2. LV systolic, diastolic, end-diastolic, dP/dt, and rate
3. PA systolic, diastolic, and mean pressure

These values are displayed in tabular form on the video monitor until a new sample is taken and stored in disc memory.

The computer samples and evaluates dilution curves for cardiac output and performs Fick-method cardiac output calculations. For the Fick method, blood gas data is required that may be entered at any time from the terminal in the monitoring room. Car-

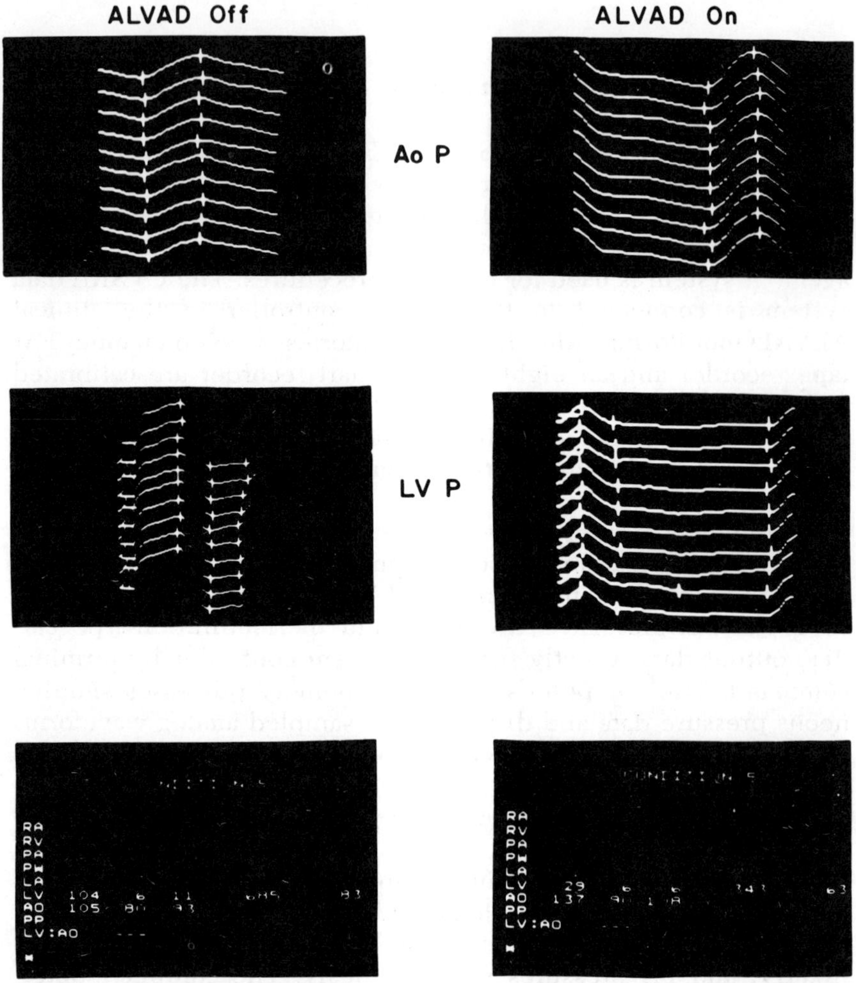

FIG. 10. Videomonitor displays of computer sampling of 10 heartbeats during failure, on and off ALVAD pump.

diac output, beat rate, and pressure data are analyzed for stroke volume, cardiac index, stroke work, and related values.

PHYSIOLOGIC DATA ACQUISITION

Arterial (radial or brachial catheter; Medicut 1002–18), pulmonary artery, pulmonary capillary wedge, and right atrial or central venous (93A-118-7F Swan-Ganz balloon-tipped catheter) pressures are monitored with Hewlett-Packard 1280C pressure transducers. Arterial pressure is continuously monitored and displayed in the operating room and ALVAD monitoring suite. Pulmonary artery pressure(s) are monitored during ALVAD assistance in the ALVAD suite.

Left ventricular pressure is monitored with an indwelling Millar PC-350 (5F) pressure transducer-tipped catheter. The catheter is inserted through a purse-string suture at the right superior pulmonary vein-left atrial juncture. The catheter and ends of the purse string are exteriorized within a 15-cm length of Teflon tubing (3-mm ID). Removal of the catheter is followed by cinching down of the purse string and buttressing with the Teflon tubing. The Teflon tubing is removed 48 hours later. Transducer outputs are coupled to a Millar TC-100 transducer control unit. Left ventricular pressure is continuously monitored and displayed in the operating room and intensive care unit. Arterial pressure (systolic/diastolic/mean; range 0 to 200 mm Hg) is obtained in the operating room with a Statham SM-1067 amplifier coupled to a Hewlett-Packard 350-1300 DC amplifier. Pressures are obtained in the ALVAD suite with a Hewlett-Packard 8805C carrier amplifier and a Hewlett-Packard 5690B cardiac catheterization computer. Computer calculation of diastolic pressure is determined by sampling each waveform for a data point at a minimal pressure level. Computer calculated systolic pressure is the maximum pressure point occurring on the waveform after assigning the diastolic pressure value. Computer calculation of mean pressure is determined mathematically by summing the value of data points for the cycle and dividing by the number of data points. All pressure data are filtered by a digital technique that removes high-frequency artifacts and catheter motion without introducing distortions into the acquired data. This is accomplished by the least squares (cubic fitting to 15 points) technique. A QRS detection unit is coupled to the analog to digital converter for reference timing purposes. Initially, 10 analog successive cycles of the pressure signal are sampled, and corresponding data points stored. The first cycle is rejected, and the resulting analyzed values are ranked for each cycle in terms of increasing magnitude. The three highest and lowest values in the series are discarded, and the values of the remaining middle third averaged. This method allows sampling and analysis of representative beats during atrial fibrillation, minimizes respiratory artifacts, and disregards premature ventricular contractions. Peak systolic left ventricular pressure (range, 0 to 200 mm Hg) is obtained in the operating room with a Hewlett-Packard 350–1100C carrier amplifier. In the ALVAD monitoring suite, peak pressures are obtained with an 8805C carrier amplifier and a 5690B cardiac catheterization computer. Mean systolic left ventricular pressure is calculated by manual planimetry.

Left ventricular end-diastolic pressure (range, 0 to 40 mm Hg) is obtained in the operating room from the left ventricular 350-1100C carrier-amplifier; attenuated, sampled manually, and logged. In the ICU, the 8805C carrier-amplifier and 5690B computer are utilized. The 8805C output is attenuated electronically with a Hewlett-Packard 8801 low-gain DC amplifier.

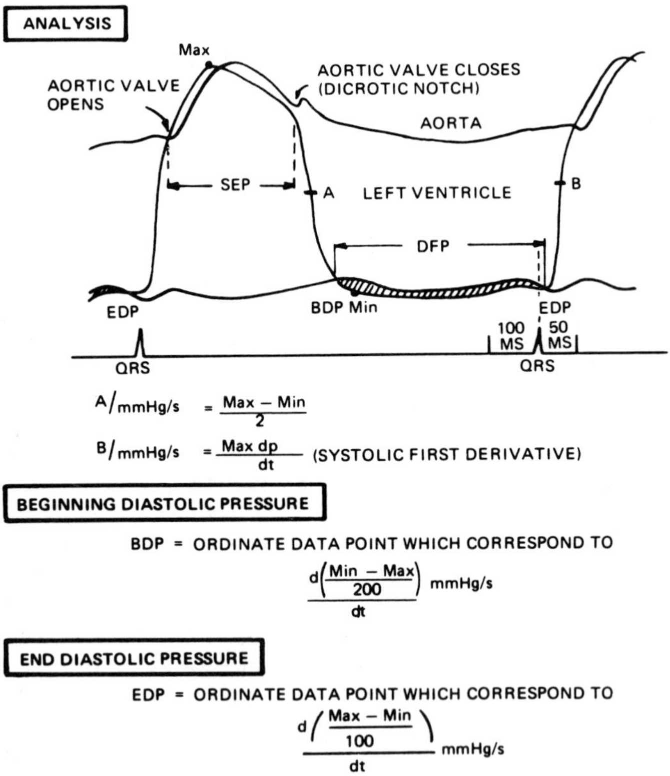

FIG. 11. Computer technique for left ventricular pressure wave form analyses.

Maximum left ventricular dP/dt (maximum first derivative of pressure with respect to time, range, 0 to ± 4000 mm Hg/sec) is obtained in the ICU with a Hewlett-Packard 8814A derivative computer and the 5690 digital computer (Fig. 11).

Pulmonary artery (systolic/diastolic/mean; range, 0 to 40 mm Hg) and pulmonary capillary wedge (mean; range, 0 to 40 mm Hg) pressure(s) are obtained with an 8805C carrier amplifier and the 5690B computer.

Right atrial or central venous (mean) pressure is obtained with an 8805C carrier amplifier and the 5690B computer (range, 0 to 40 mm Hg) or a water manometer (range, 0 to 55 cm H_2O).

The electrocardiogram is obtained in the operating room with a Statham SM-1066 amplifier coupled to a Hewlett-Packard 350-1300 DC amplifier, continuously displayed and monitored. Heart rate is calculated manually with the formula: HR = 60 C/L, where HR = heart rate (B/min), C = paper speed (mm/sec), and L = R-R interval length (mm). In the ICU, the electrocardiogram is obtained with a Hewlett-Packard 8811B amplifier. Heart rate is obtained from the 5690B computer, which uses the formula: HR = (1000/Ls) × 60, where Ls = left ventricular peak systolic to peak systolic interval time (msec).

Cardiac output is calculated by one of three methods: (a) indicator dilution (green dye); (b) thermodilution (using a 93A-118-7F Swan-Ganz balloon-tipped catheter with thermistor tip); or (c) digital readout from the pneumatic pump monitor (during total ALVAD assistance).

The indicator dilution (green dye) technique (Hamilton formula) is performed on-line and displayed instantaneously with the 5690B computer, using the formula:

$$CO = \frac{I}{\bar{c} \times t} \times 60$$

where CO = cardiac output (liters/minute), I = amount of indicator injected (mg), $\bar{c}$ = mean indicator concentration for first circulation (mg/liter), and t = time for first circulation (sec). To obviate the problem of dye recirculation (required for mean indicator concentration calculation), a computer pattern recognition program (Fig. 12) employs points on the curve downslope between 0.6 and 0.4 of the maximum height. The 5691A computer keyboard is used to initiate the calibration and calculation of the dye curve.

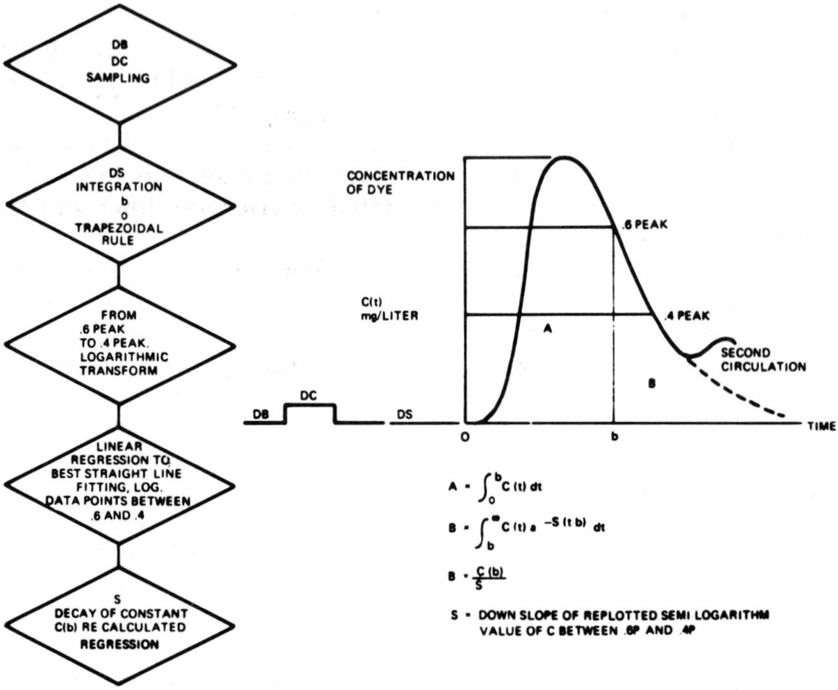

$$A = \int_0^b C(t)\,dt$$

$$B = \int_b^\infty C(t)\,e^{-S(t\,b)}\,dt$$

$$B = \frac{C(b)}{S}$$

FIG. 12. Computer technique for dye dilution cardiac output analyses (using Hamilton Formula).

The dye baseline key is used to record the densitometer zero baseline (dye-free blood sample). The dye calibration key is used to record the densitometer calibration factor (known dye concentration blood sample). The first portion of the dye curve is integrated by the computer, using trapezoidal integration (sampling rate 10 points/sec). Data points sampled from 60 to 40 percent of the peak curve (downslope) are transformed into logarithmic values. A least square linear regression is performed to assure a linear variation of the data points logarithm. The first derivative of the linear regression line is measured and used to calculate the remaining curve contour. The dye curve and calculated cardiac output are displayed on the 5651 video monitor in the ALVAD monitoring suite; cardiac output values are computer-stored for later retrieval. For cardiac output determinations, 5 to 10 mg of indocyanine green dye are injected into the right atrium (via a Swan-Ganz catheter) with arterial withdrawal (radial or brachial catheter) through a Gilson densitometer. Cardiac index is calculated by the 5690B computer with the formula: CI (liters/minute/meter²) = CO (liters/minute)/BSA (meter²).

The dye dilution technique requires withdrawal of arterial blood during measurements and removal of blood for calibration. In addition, the validity of the method in low-output states may be questioned because of early dye recirculation. The use of heat as an indicator (thermodilution) eliminates most of these problems in normothermic patients. Withdrawal of blood is not needed because the temperature of blood and its changes following injection of a cold liquid into the right atrium are measured by a thermistor in the pulmonary artery (93A-118-7F Swan-Ganz balloon-tipped catheter with thermistor tip). The catheter has two small and two large lumens. One large lumen terminates at the tip and serves for monitoring pulmonary artery and pulmonary capillary wedge pressure(s). The second large lumen terminates about 30 cm proximal to the tip and is used for injection of cold liquid into the right atrium or superior vena cava and for pressure measurements. One small lumen allows inflation and deflation of the balloon, fastened 1 to 2 mm from the tip. The second small lumen contains the thermistor leads, mounted on the catheter surface just proximal to the balloon. The temperature-time curve is calibrated, in situ, by a resistance, which represents a temperature difference, known from the temperature-resistance relationship of the thermistor. Five milliliters of cold (0 to 5 C) 5 percent dextrose solution is injected rapidly via the proximal lumen into the right atrium or superior vena cava. The off-balance output of the thermistor bridge, resulting from the change in blood temperature, is amplified and recorded. Thermodilution cardiac outputs are obtained using an Edwards Laboratory Model 9510 Cardiac Output Computer, which uses the formula:

$$CO = \frac{1.08\ Ct(60)\ V_I(T_B - T_I)}{\int_0^t T_B(t)\ dt}$$

where 1.08 = pCp [5 percent dextrose]/pCp [blood] (p = density, Cp = specific heat), Ct = correction for injectate temperature rise, 60 = sec/minute, V_I = volume of injectate (ml), T_B = initial blood temperature (C), T_I = initial injectate temperature (C) and $\int_0^t T_B(t)$ = integral of blood temperature change (C sec). Cardiac output determinations are entered into the 5690B computer off-line.

In addition, during total ALVAD assistance, the cardiac output is obtained from the pneumatic pump monitor. These outputs can be measured only during on-pump conditions. The piston displacement and driveline pressure signals from the pneumatic pump monitor are utilized to compute stroke volume with the formula:

$$SV = ApX - V_1 \frac{P_T}{P_{atm} + P_T}$$

where SV = stroke volume (ml/B), Ap = piston area (cm^2), X = piston displacement (cm), V_1 = initial air volume within the isolation cylinder, driveline, and pump housing (ml), P_T = driveline pressure (mm Hg), and P_{atm} = atmospheric pressure (mm Hg). The computed stroke volume is multiplied by the rate to yield cardiac output. Stroke volumes, rates, and minute outputs are available as digital readouts from the pneumatic pump monitor. Cardiac output calculations are entered into the 5690B computer off-line.

Left ventricular stroke-work index is obtained with the 5690B computer or calculated manually, using the formula:

$$SWI = \frac{LVP_{sm}\,(13.6\ CI)}{HR}$$

where SWI = left ventricular stroke work index (normal range, 50 to 85 gm meter/beat/meter^2), LVP_{sm} = left ventricular mean systolic pressure [(mm Hg) computer calculated but not displayed], CI = cardiac index (liters/minute/meter^2), 13.6 = conversion factor from mm Hg cm^3 to gm meter, and HR = heart rate (beats/minute).

Total systemic vascular resistance is obtained with the 5690B computer or calculated manually using the formula:

$$SVR = \frac{AoP_m - RA_m}{CO}$$

where SVR = total systemic vascular resistance [normal range 12.0-16.0 resistance units; mm Hg/(liters/minute)], AoP_m = mean arterial pressure (mm Hg), RA_m = mean right atrial pressure (mm Hg), and CO = cardiac output (liters/minute). Derivation of absolute resistance is made by multiplying SVR by the conversion factor of 80 [1 mm Hg/(liters/minute) = 80 dynes sec cm^{-5}; normal range, 950 to 1300].

Pulmonary arteriolar resistance is obtained with the 5690B computer or calculated manually, using the formula:

$$PAR = \frac{PA_m - PCW_m}{CO}$$

where PAR = pulmonary arteriolar resistance [normal range, 0.5 to 1.0 resistance units; mm Hg (liters/minute)], PA_m = mean pulmonary artery pressure (mm Hg), PCW_m = mean pulmonary capillary wedge pressure (mm Hg), and CO = cardiac output (liters/minute). Derivation of absolute resistance is made by multiplying PAR by the conversion factor of 80 [1 mm Hg/liters/minute) = 80 dynes sec cm^{-5}; normal range, 40 to 90].

Left ventricular tension time index [pressure rate product (index of myocardial oxygen demand), normal range 2000 to 3000 mm Hg sec/minute] is calculated manually using the formula:

$$TTI = \overline{LVP}_s \times SP \times HR$$

where TTI = left ventricular tension time index (mm Hg sec/minute), $\overline{LVP}_s$ = left ventricular mean systolic pressure (mm Hg), SP = left ventricular systolic time (interval from beginning of systolic pressure rise to beginning of diastole measured in seconds), and HR = heart rate (beats/minute).

Left ventricular diastolic pressure time index (index of myocardial oxygen supply; normal range, 2500 to 3500 mm Hg sec/minute) is computed using the formula:

$$DPTI = (AoP_{md} - LVDP_m) \times DP \times HR$$

where DPTI = left ventricular diastolic pressure time index (mm Hg sec/minute), AoP_{md} = mean diastolic arterial pressure (mm Hg), $LVDP_m$ = left ventricular mean diastolic pressure (mm Hg), DP = left ventricular diastolic time (interval from beginning of diastole to beginning systolic pressure rise measured in seconds), and HR = heart rate (beats/minute). The index of myocardial oxygen supply/demand is calculated by dividing DPTI by TTI (normal range, 0.9 to 1.5).*

Left ventricular echocardiography is performed following ALVAD implantation. The ultrasonic measurements are obtained

**Datascope EVR Computer Model No. 0400-0000.*

using a Unirad 100 Series Echoscope with Cambridge Multichannel Recorder. A 5.0 MHz, 3.5 MHz, or 2.25 MHz transducer (focused at 5 cm) is utilized. Each has an active crystal diameter of 3/16 inch and an outer diameter of 1/4 inch. Echocardiograms are recorded on Polaroid film or photographic paper. With the patient in the supine position, the transducer is positioned along the left sternal border in the third to fifth intercostal space (position for maximum anterior mitral valve echo). From this position, the transducer is rotated so that prominent endocardial echos from the left ventricular free wall and septum are recorded. In order to obtain the lateral minor dimension of the cavity perpendicular to the major axis, the ventricle is scanned inferiorly and superiorly along the major axis, until echoes corresponding to the anterior and posterior mitral valve are visualized (Fig. 13).

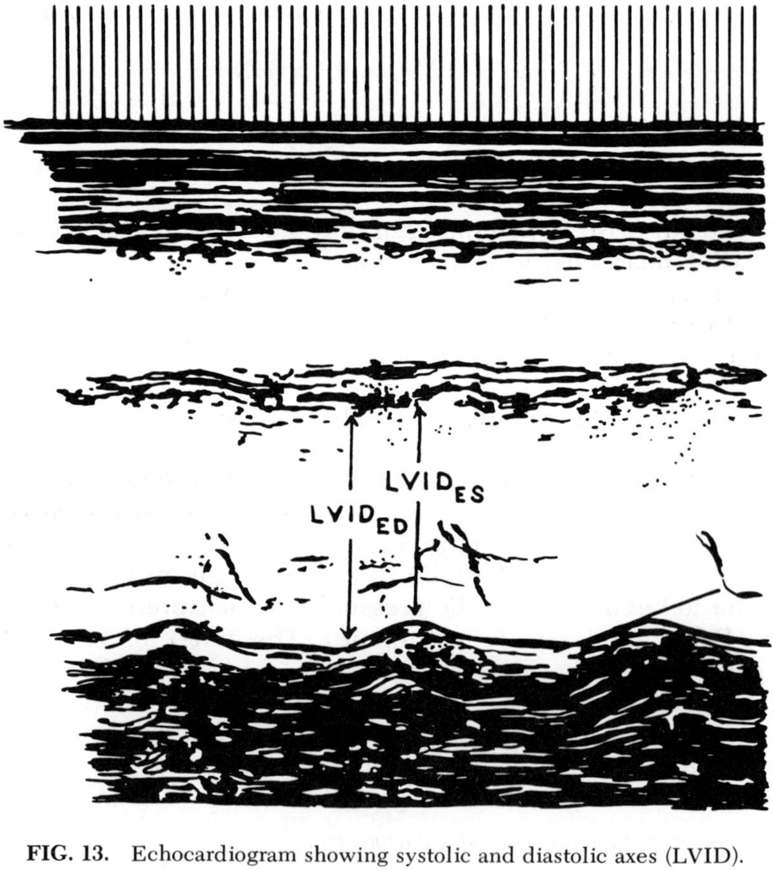

FIG. 13. Echocardiogram showing systolic and diastolic axes (LVID).

Left ventricular end-diastolic volume is obtained with the H-P 9810A programmable calculator, using the curvilinear regression formula:

$$\text{LVEDV echo} = 14.6\ \text{LVID} + 0.62\ (\text{LVID}^3) - 19.1$$

where LVEDV echo = left ventricular end-diastolic volume (normal range, 100 to 140 ml); 14.6, 0.62, and 19.1 = regression equation constants; and LVID = left ventricular internal diameter (measured in cm as the minor axis distance between the left septal echo and LV endocardial echo in end-diastole). Bulging of the minor dimension (LVID) during isovolumic systole (manifested by a posterior movement of the endocardium) is compensated for by calculating LVID at the onset of the Q wave of the EKG rather than the R wave. This curvilinear regression equation is utilized for LVID measurements ranging from 2 to 8 cm (15 to 415 ml EDV).

Left ventricular end-systolic volume (normal range, 25 to 60 ml) is obtained with the 9810A programmable calculator, using the formula:

$$\text{LVESV} = \text{LVEDV echo} - \text{SV}$$

where LVESV = left ventricular end-systolic volume (ml), LVEDV echo = left ventricular end-diastolic volume (ml; obtained echocardiographically), and SV = left ventricular stroke volume (calculated from the indicator dilution, thermodilution, or pneumatic pump monitor display cardiac output value divided by the heart rate).

Left ventricular ejection fraction (normal range, 0.60 to 0.70) is obtained with the 9810A calculator, using the formula:

$$\text{EF} = \text{SV/LVEDV echo}$$

where EF = left ventricular ejection fraction; SV and LVEDV echo measurements are calculator-stored and are recalled for LVESV determinations.

CURRENT ACTIVITIES

Since November 1, 1975, the instrumentation, facilities, and supporting personnel described in the foregoing sections have been maintained in readiness in our institutions. Because the clinical investigative protocol is extensive, categorically rigorous, and restrictive, every clinical effort has been made to avoid situations wherein the ALVAD becomes the only viable option. Nonetheless, when such discrete, defined situations have arisen and the ALVAD was utilized, the same degree of effort has been exerted to document in detail any technical, mechanical, ethical, legal, or social misadventures.* ALVAD units are maintained in a sterile state, the clinical console is tested throughout all of its design capabilities each week, and the computerized monitoring system is used routinely during each clinical situation wherein IABP alone is needed. The clinical engineering members of the group have designed, assembled, and utilized all of the instrumentation connecting the ALVAD suite to the laboratories and worked in each of the operating rooms.

A description of the clinical protocol is beyond the scope of this report. It is available on request. Between November 1, 1975 and April 15, 1976 (a 5.5-month period), 1483 adult patients underwent procedures requiring cardiopulmonary bypass in our facilities. Eighty-nine percent (1327) were weaned from bypass, uneventfully. Seventy-one percent (1062) developed normotensive arterial pressures and recovered uneventfully; 265 (17.9 percent) had hypotension and low cardiac output within the first 24 hours following cardiopulmonary bypass. Of these, 244 (16.5 percent) had adequate responses to pharmacologic or IABP therapy, and recovered. Twenty-one (1.4 percent) had inadequate responses to pharmacologic or IABP therapy. The ALVAD was not employed, and all expired.

One hundred and forty-seven patients (10 percent) were not weaned from cardiopulmonary bypass uneventfully. One hundred and eighteen (7.9 percent) had adequate responses to pharmacologic therapy according to the NHLI protocol, and recovered. Twenty-nine patients (2 percent) had inadequate responses to pharmacologic measures. Fifteen (1 percent) had inadequate responses to IABP; 13 (0.9 percent) did not receive ALVAD assistance, and all expired. Two (0.1 percent) expired despite preterminal ALVAD assistance. Eight (0.5 percent) had adequate responses to IABP, and recovered. Six (0.4 percent) did not receive IABP assistance; five (0.3 percent) did not receive ALVAD assistance, and expired. One (0.1 percent) expired despite ALVAD

**THI Clinical ALVAD Reports to NHLI, January 13, 1976; February 8, 1976; March 15, 1976; and May 28, 1976.*

assistance. Nine patients (1 percent) sustained intraoperative complications, unrelated to cardiopulmonary bypass; all expired.

These data are summarized in the matrix in Figure 14. Stated more succinctly: 1483 patients underwent procedures requiring cardiopulmonary bypass in a 5.5-month period. Fifty-one (3.4 percent) died within 48 hours. Thirty-six (2.4 percent) received IABP assistance by our Circulatory Support Services, and eleven survived. Fifteen patients were identified as ALVAD candidates according to our rigorous institutional and federal protocols. Three (0.2 percent) underwent partial artificial heart (ALVAD) implantation. In retrospect, twelve others fulfilled the criteria but did not undergo ALVAD implantation.

As of this writing, four patients have undergone ALVAD implantation. All were male, with age ranges between 47 and 58 years. Their diagnoses, operative procedures, pre- or postoperative use of the less effective IABP prior to ALVAD implantation, the ALVAD-generated flows achieved, and duration of ALVAD assistance are summarized in Table 1. The hemodynamic effectiveness of various left ventricular assist devices is summarized in Table 2.

INITIAL CLINICAL OBSERVATIONS AND EVOLVING CONCEPTS

A number of preliminary observations and tentative concepts have been recorded and formulated from this early experience, ie, broadly, the aura and mystique of artificial hearts can be gradually dispelled along with their casual association with laboratory gadgetry. Reduced to their least common denominators, they are simply intracorporeal blood pumps, designed and tested to be compatible with all body components. The ALVAD is an intracorporeal auxiliary left ventricle that can perform in excess of 80 percent of the total work of the heart. Many of our experimental investigations have, in the main, centered on the physiologic effects of "resting" the biologic left ventricle by such biocompatible, mechanical means. Some of these studies are summarized in Tables 3–7. Concomitantly and equally important, these initial clinical trials have demonstrated that the legal, moral, ethical, and social implications of partial artificial hearts are vastly overstated and, in general, surrounded by a fear of the unknown. Given a reasonable, thoughtful, and compassionate explanation, including risk/benefit ratios in desperate circumstances, all families and pa-

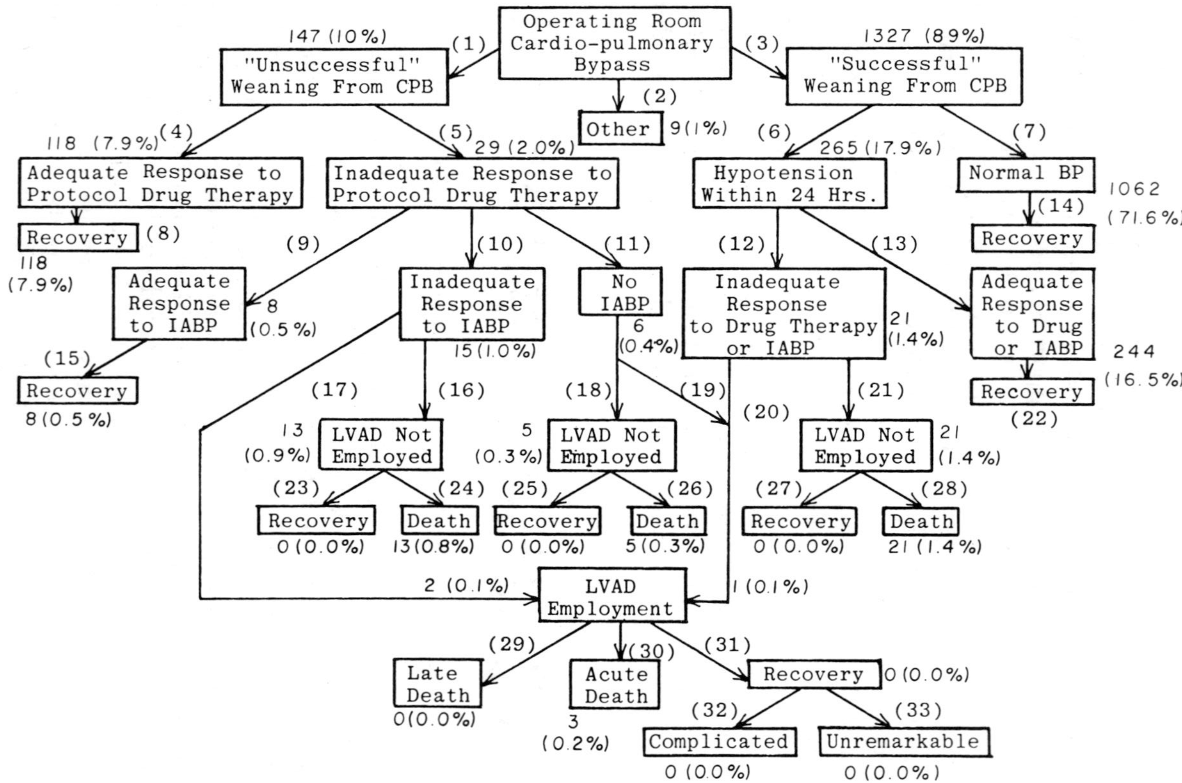

FIG. 14. THI-ALVAD Patient Entry Matrix: 1483 patients analyzed in 5.5-month period (November 1, 1975–April 15, 1976).

TABLE 1. Initial Alvad Clinical Trials THI 1975–76*

AGE, SEX	DIAGNOSIS	DATE	PROCEDURE	IABP	ALVAD	ALVAD Q (LITERS/MIN)	DURATION (HRS)
58, M	AMI, Dec 1975, CAOD, (LAD-diagonal) LV failure Pul. Edema	12-23-75	ACB (LAD) Chronic infarctectomy	Preop 12-19-75	Postop 12-23-75	3, during V-tachycardia V.-fibrillation	1
52, M	AMI, Dec 1975, CAOD, (Right, LAD, proximal Cx, and OM[1])	2-4-76	ACB [Right (PD), LAD, and OM[1]]	Postop 2-4-76	Postop 2-4-76	4	2
61, M	Preinfarction angina CAOD (Right, left main, LAD, diagonal and proximal Cx). Arrest during diagnostic catheterization	3-4-76	External massage FV-FA bypass with oxygenation. ACB (LAD and OM[1])	Postop 3-4-76	Postop 3-4-76	3.5	3
47, M	RHD, AI, MI, CHF, LVH, LAHB, Low CO	5-19-76	MVR, AVR	—	Postop 5-19-76	3.5	8
44, F	Angina CAOD (Right, LAD, Cx)	6-30-76	ACB (Right, LAD), LAD endarterectomy	Postop 7-5-76	Postop 6-30-76	4	140

**Key:* *AMI: acute myocardiaol infarction; CAOD: coronary artery occlusive disease; LAHB: left anterior hemiblock; LAD: left anterior descending; RHD: rheumatic heart disease; AI: aortic insufficiency; CHF: congestive heart failure; LVH: left ventricular hypertrophy; MVR: mitral valve replacement; AVR: aortic valve replacement; OM[1]: first obtuse marginal.*

TABLE 2. Summary of Hemodynamic Effectiveness of Various Left Ventricular Assist Devices*

HEMODYNAMIC VARIABLE	IABP (MGH)	ROLLER PUMP (LA-Ao) (PENN)	ROLLER PUMP (LV-Ao) (PENN)	ALVAD (LV-Ao) (THI)	EFFECTIVENESS ALVAD/IABP
LV peak systolic pressure	↓9	↓14	↓96	↓88	9.8
LV stroke work	↓20	↓82	↓100	↓84	4.2
LV dP/dt	↓1	↓28	↓80	↓83	83.0
Coronary sinus flow	↓7	↓16	↓42	↓25	3.6
Myocardial oxygen consumption	↓13	↓22	↓47	↓40	3.1

**Based on studies done at the Massachusetts General Hospital, Pennsylvania State University Hospital, and Texas Heart Institute. All values in the first four columns are percentages. IABP: intra-aortic balloon pumping; LA: left atrium; Ao: aorta; LV: left ventricle; ALVAD: abdominal left ventricular assist device; dP/dt: rate of pressure rise.*

TABLE 3. Effects of Abdominal Left Ventricular Assist Device (ALVAD) Pumping: Summary*

PARAMETER	ALVAD EFFECT
Aortic pressure (systolic)	↑27%
Aortic pressure (diastolic)	↑13%
Aortic pressure (mean)	↑18%
Peak LV pressure	↓88%
LV end-diastolic pressure	↓33%
LV tension-time index	↓83%
LV dP/dt	↓96%
A-VO_2 difference	↓20%
Coronary blood flow	↓19%
Myocardial oxygen consumption	↓34%

**Acute canine studies (nonischemic heart). These acute canine studies demonstrate the effects of ALVAD pumping on maintaining systemic perfusion while lowering left ventrciular work, oxygen consumption, and coronary blood flow.*

tients have agreed in the presence of their advocates that such courses should be attempted.

Nonetheless, at this very early phase of our knowledge, our legal advisors strongly suggest the obtaining of prior informed consent. The current federally approved protocol is quite restric-

TABLE 4. Effects of Abdominal Left Ventricular Assist Device (ALVAD) Pumping: Summary*

PARAMETER	ALVAD EFFECT
LV end-diastolic pressure	↓59%
Coronary perfusion pressure	↑31%
LV dP/dt	↓79%
Peak LV wall tension	↓80%
LV stroke work	↓78%
LV pressure-time product	↓84%
LV end-diastolic volume	↓39%
LV end-systolic volume	↓69%
LV stroke volume	↑23%
Cardiac output	↑21%
Ejection fraction	↑77%

**Acute canine studies (ischemic heart). These studies demonstrate the effects of ALVAD pumping during periods of induced myocardial ischemia. Systemic perfusion is increased while left ventricular work is reduced; ejection fraction is increased. Ventricular dilatation (end-diastolic pressure and volume) is reduced during ALVAD pumping.*

TABLE 5. Effects of Abdominal Left Ventricular Assist Device (ALVAD) Pumping: Summary*

PARAMETER	ALVAD EFFECT
Aortic pressure (mean)	↑16%
LV pressure (mean systolic)	↓88%
LV end-diastolic pressure	↓62%
Heart rate	↓4%
RV stroke volume	↑16%
Peak RV pressure	↓2%
RV end-diastolic pressure	↓8%
Cardiac output	↑13%
LV stroke work	↓90%
Tension time index (TTI)	↓70%
Diastolic pressure time index (DPTI)	↑28%
DPTI/TTI	↑426%
Coronary blood flow	↓33%

**Acute bovine studies (nonischemic heart). These studies demonstrate the effects of ALVAD pumping on maintaining systemic perfusion while lowering left ventricular work and coronary blood flow. The myocardial oxygen supply/demand ratio (DPTI/TTI) is increased four-fold during ALVAD pumping.*

TABLE 6. Effects of Abdominal Left Ventricular Assist Device (ALVAD) Pumping: Summary*

PARAMETER	ALVAD EFFECT
Aortic pressure (mean)	↑44%
LV pressure (mean systolic)	↓91%
LV end-diastolic pressure	↓80%
Heart rate	↓5%
RV stroke volume	↑24%
Cardiac output	↑18%
LV stroke work	↓93%
Tension time index (TTI)	↓81%
Diastolic pressure time index (DPTI)	↑82%
DPTI/TTI	↑896%

**Acute bovine studies (ischemic heart). These acute bovine studies demonstrate the effects of ALVAD pumping during periods of induced myocardial ischemia. Systemic perfusion is increased while left ventricular work is reduced. Myocardial oxygen supply/demand ratio (TTI/DPTI) is increased eight-fold during ALVAD pumping.*

TABLE 7. Effects of Abdominal Left Ventricular Assist Device (ALVAD) Pumping: Summary*

PARAMETER	ALVAD EFFECT
Aortic pressure (systolic)	↑11%
Aortic pressure (diastolic)	↓2%
Aortic pressure (mean)	↑4%
LV pressure (mean systolic)	↓42%
LV end-diastolic pressure	↓34%
LV dP/dt	↓46%
Heart rate	↓6%
Cardiac output	↑4%
LV pressure-rate product	↓45%
LV stroke work	↓47%
% cardiac output assumed by ALVAD	97 ± 7%

**Chronic bovine studies. These chronic bovine studies demonstrate the effects of ALVAD pumping on chronically maintaining systemic perfusion while lowering left ventricular work. The ALVAD chronically assumed 97±7% of the cardiac output while lowering LV stroke work nearly 50% over periods up to one month.*

tive in assuring a preterminal state. At this stage, scrupulous adherence to its guidelines and intricacies is mandatory.

The technical aspects of clinical ALVAD implantation require more than the usual attention to hemeostasis, in all areas, in these totally heparinized patients on prolonged cardiopulmonary bypass. In addition, the anastomosis of the outlet graft to the abdominal aorta requires more than the usual vascular surgical attention, because it is subjected to ALVAD-generated pressures, which can exceed 150 mm Hg. Mention should also be made regarding the methods of attaching the inlet sewing ring to the left ventricular apex. It would seem that this is most expeditiously accomplished by coring the apex first, after cross-clamping the ascending aorta, stabilizing the heart with the operator's index and third fingers within the left ventricle, and suturing the sewing ring with circumferential, individual, double-armed mattress sutures of 2-0 Tycron, buttressed with Teflon pledgets. Following pump implantation, the ascending aorta and outlet graft cross-clamps should not be released until the ALVAD has been actuated for a stroke or two, and any residual air evacuated or aspirated, proximally from the ascending aorta and distally from the outlet graft.

The pump has functioned well in man, as it has in our extended series of bovine experiments, and is capable of generating near-adequate flows in the presence of ventricular fibrillation. A representative tracing is shown in Figure 15. A roentgenogram of the unit in situ, in mechanical systole, in man, is shown in Figure 16. Because the ALVAD is capable of totally unloading the left ventricle for periods up to one month, it is not unreasonable to predict that with further, careful, conservative evaluations, the potential of allowing the human left ventricle to rest for prolonged periods will be gradually realized.

SUMMARY

An intracorporeal left ventricular assist device has been designed, developed, modified, tested in vitro and in vivo, validated, and approved by federal auspices for initial, controlled clinical trials in our institutions. These trials are being undertaken according to a rigorous protocol that precludes premature use and facilitates careful documentation. These efforts are the result of nearly a decade of NHI-NHLI sponsored R&D. The ALVAD is pneumatically actuated by an external console with multiple failsafe subsystems. Its physiologic effectiveness in profound unloading of the left ventricle, mechanical durability and reliability, biocompatibility, patient-acceptability, and need in our patient population, have been the subject of six federal reviews by extramural Ad Hoc committees drawn from experts in the involved

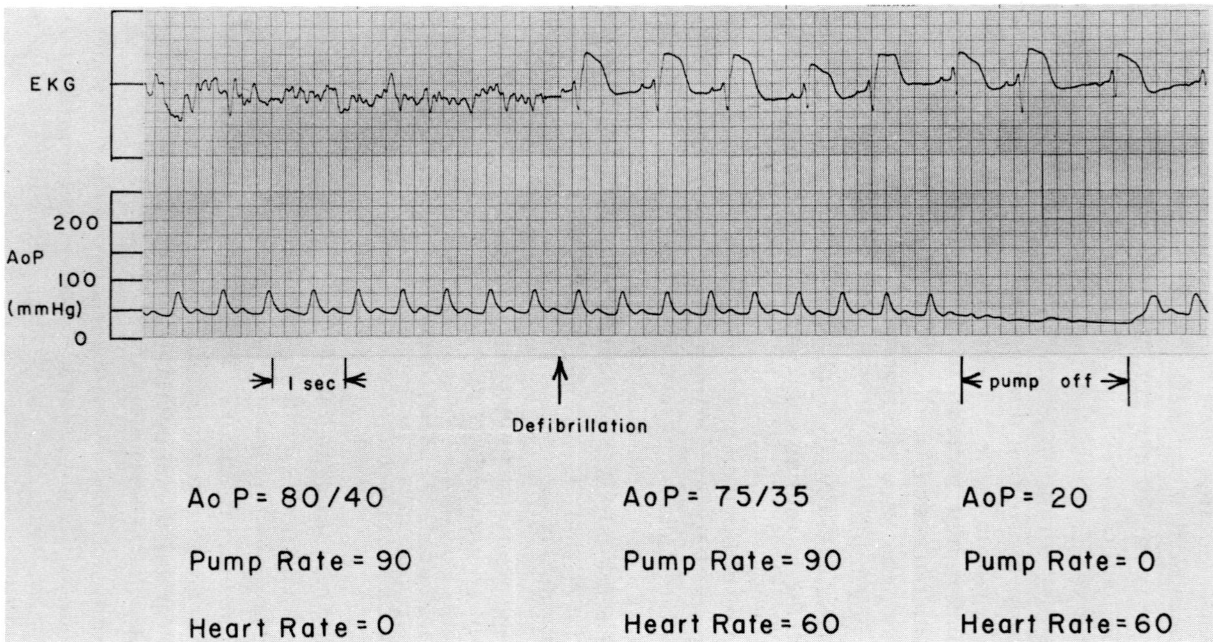

FIG. 15. ALVAD actuation in man during ventricular fibrillation, defibrillation and without ALVAD for approximately two seconds.

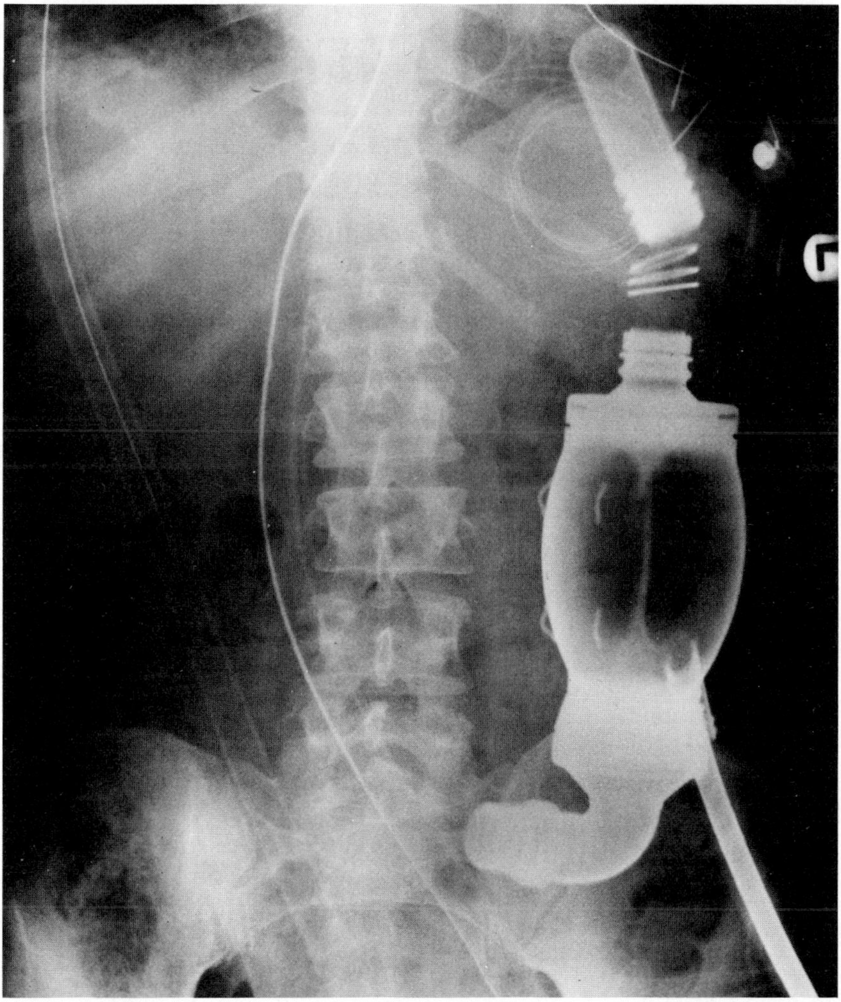

FIG. 16. Roentgenogram of the abdomen with the intracorporeal ALVAD in situ, in mechanical systole, in man.

disciplines. The legal, moral, ethical, and social implications of its use in man have been given similar in-depth considerations by similar committees. It had been implanted in 200 or more experimental animals for periods up to two times that of its intended period of use (14 days-1 month), prior to the first clinical trial on December 23, 1975. Unlike the intra-aortic balloon pump, which augments existing circulation, or extracorporeal left atrial-to-systemic pumping systems, the ALVAD is a true intracorporeal blood pump, 6 to 10 times more effective, and a prototype of more sophisticated, longer-lived electrical or nuclear-actuated devices still under development. It can operate independent of an intact EKG signal, and is capable of generating flows up to 10 liters/minute. It cannot, however, substitute for right heart function, and pumps only what it receives. Its clinical state-of-the-art can be likened to that of IABP augmentation of a decade ago and cardiopulmonary bypass of two decades ago.

Thus far, four adult male patients have been studied (see Addendum). Prior informed consent was obtained from each patient or his nearest relative. No difficulties have been encountered during implantation, although special precautions have been taken to insure blood and air-tight anastomoses at the infrarenal abdominal aorta and left ventricular apex exit and entry sites. The pump has performed in man as it has in our extended series of animal experiments, achieving flows of 3 to 4.5 liters/minute. No evidence of excessive hemolysis, embolic phenomena, or visceral encroachment has been encountered. The outlet graft has been modified and is now a low-porosity component, freshly preclotted. Thus far, because of ethical considerations, each clinical implantation has been undertaken in essentially moribund patients, maintained with cardiopulmonary bypass and IABP. The pump is capable of producing an adequate circulation in the presence of ventricular fibrillation or standstill.

In our view, the device deserves controlled clinical evaluations in less desperate circumstances, at earlier periods of left ventricular deterioration, in the presence of intact right heart function following inability to wean from cardiopulmonary bypass. Its possible application in other low-output states, eg, postinfarction, profound cardiogenic shock, deserves parallel preliminary consideration.

ADDENDUM

Since this report was submitted, this intracorporeal partial artificial heart (ALVAD) was utilized in a fifth patient, a 44-year-old female. Her pre-operative diagnosis was coronary artery occlusive disease involving three vessels, and she underwent a double reversed saphenous vein aorto-coronary bypass procedure to the right and left anterior descending coronary arteries with endarterectomy of the latter. Following the procedure, the patient could not be weaned from cardiopulmonary bypass, and exhibited no ventricular ejection with intermittent asystole, electromechanical dissociation and episodes of persistent ventricular fibrillation. Because of her terminal condition, the ALVAD was implanted and ventricular function returned over the next six days during total left ventricular unloading. On the fifth to sixth postoperative days, the patient was weaned from ALVAD support to intra-aortic balloon pumping (IABP). The ALVAD was removed on the sixth postoperative day without incident.

Oliguria progressing to anuria beginning on the first post-ALVAD implant day required multiple hemodialyses. Renal failure continued to be a problem and was the ultimate cause of the patient's death 12 days after implantation and seven days after weaning from ALVAD to IABP on the 12th postoperative day. The details of this first hemodynamically successful use of this intracorporeal left ventricular assist device have been reported to the Artificial Heart Program Office.[3–5]

REFERENCES

1. NHLI: Criteria for Clinical Investigative Use of Left Ventricular Assist Devices, Aug. 8, 1974, sec. III, c 3
2. Norman JC, Bernhard WF: Criteria, protocols and reporting forms for initial left ventricular assist device clinical trials. Cardiovascular Diseases Bull THI 2(Suppl):438, 1975
3. THI Clinical ALVAD Report to NHLI #5, July 12, 1976
4. Norman JC: The Clinical Applications of Left Ventricular Assist Devices (ALVAD) Contract Number NO1-HV-5-3006, Report Number NO1-HV-5-3006-1, July 4, 1976 pp 1–239
5. Norman JC: Hemodynamic Effects of ALVAD Pumping in Man. Topical Report to NHLB (Contract Number NO1-HV-5-3006-2, July 28, 1976, pp 1–36

BIBLIOGRAPHY

Aldrich JG, Chambers JA, Daly BDT, et al: A totally implantable electrically actuated left ventricular assist device (LVAD): In-vivo testing. Proc of 26th Ann Conf on Eng and Med in Biol 15:330, 1973

Arthur J, Dove GB, Migliore JJ, et al: A comparison of acute hemodynamic effects of abdominal left ventricular assist device (ALVAD) pumping in the nonfailing and failing canine heart. Clin Res 21(3):401, 1973

Carlos CJ, Daly B, Migliore J, et al: Improved design and experimental management modifications in abdominal left ventricular assist device: Preclinical testing. Medical Instrumentation 9(1):66, 1975

Carlos CJ, Edmonds CH, Fuqua JM, et al: Production of controlled reversible left ventricular failure in calves using intracoronary lidocaine hydrochloride: A useful method of evaluating left ventricular assist devices. Ann Thorac Surg 21(3):209, 1976

Carlos CJ, Igo SR, Hibbs C, et al: Controlled production of left ventricular failure in open and closed chest calves using intracoronary lidocaine hydrochloride (xylocaine). Amer Soc Artif Intern Organs Abstracts 4:8, 1975

Carlos CJ, Igo SR, Hibbs CW, Nitta S, Norman JC: Physiologic effects of varying degrees of afterloading with levarterenol and nitroprusside during abdominal left ventricular assist device (ALVAD) pumping in the awake, anesthetized calf. Amer Soc Artif Intern Organs Abstracts 4:8, 1975

Carlos CJ, Nitta S, Igo SR, Norman JC: Abdominal left ventricular assist device (ALVAD): Hemodynamic effects after lidocaine-induced left ventricular failure. Proc 28th Ann Conf on Eng in Med and Biol 17:358, 1975

Daly BDT, Edmonds CH, Igo SR, et al: Right ventricular effects of left ventricular unloading with an abdominal left ventricular assist device (ALVAD) in the calf. The Physiologist 17(3):205, 1974

Daly BDT, Migliore JJ, Norman JC: Ventilatory management of calves undergoing thoracotomy. Clin Res 21(3):412, 1972

Daly BDT, Migliore JJ, Robinson WJ, O'Brien JW, Norman JC: Respiratory support during experimental circulatory support systems implantation. Clin Res 20(5):855, 1972

Dove GB, Arthur J, Migliore JJ, et al: End-diastolic segment length (EDSL) and derived muscle length (ML) analyses during abdominal left ventricular assist device (ALVAD) pumping (abstract). Clin Res 21(3):415, 1973

Dove GB, Migliore JJ, Fuqua JM, et al: An abdominal left ventricular assist device (ALVAD): Experimental physiologic analyses, III. Cardiac output. Proc of 26th Ann Conf on Eng in Med and Biol 15:148, 1973

Edmonds CH, Fuqua JM, Carlos CJ, Norman JC: Effects of increasing preload during abdominal left ventricular assist device (ALVAD) pumping. Proc 28th Ann Conf on Eng in Med and Biol 17:357, 1975

Edmonds CH, Fuqua JM, McMillan MK, Migliore JJ, Norman JC: The effects of an abdominal left ventricular assist device on erythrocyte osmotic fragility. Medical Instrumentation 9(1):67, 1975

Edmonds CH, Hughes DA, Fuqua JM, et al: Hematologic, biochemical and coagulation values in the normal Hereford calf. Amer Soc Artif Intern Organs Abstracts 3:20, 1974

Edmonds CH, Igo SR, Huffman FN, Norman JC: Effects of blood pump inflow tubes retained in the left ventricular apex. Amer Soc Artif Intern Organs Abstracts 3:21, 1974

Edmonds CH, McMillan MK, Wheeler NW, Austin SF, Norman JC: Postoperative transfusion therapy in calves. Amer Soc Artif Intern Organs Abstracts 5:23, 1976

Edmonds CH, Naifeh J, Walker M, et al: Documentation of clinical readiness of an abdominal left ventricular assist device (ALVAD). Amer Soc Artif Intern Organs Abstracts 5:23, 1976

Fuqua JM, Edmonds CH, Carlos CJ, Norman JC: An intracorporeal left ventricular assist device: Human fitting studies. Amer Soc Artif Intern Organs Abstracts 4:19, 1975

Fuqua JM, Hibbs C, Thompson P, et al: Performance of an abdominal left ventricular assist device (ALVAD) during simulated tachycardias and dysrhythmias in the calf. Medical Instrumentation 10(1):56, 1976

Fuqua JM, Igo SR, Edmonds CH, et al: An abdominal left ventricular assist device: Experimental physiologic analyses, V. Clin Res 22(1):5A, 1974

Galioto FM, Dawson JT, Migliore JJ, et al: Serial echocardiographic assessment of left ventricular function in the calf before and after abdominal left ventricular assist device implantation. FASEB 32(3):332, 1973

Hibbs CW, Fuqua JM, Robinson WJ, Norman JC: Computerized monitoring system for clinical left ventricular assist device evaluations. Proc 28th Ann Conf on Eng in Med and Biol 17:356, 1975

Hibbs CW, Fuqua JM, Robinson WJ, Norman JC: Deleterious effects of improper synchronization during implantable left ventricular assist pumping. Amer Soc Artif Intern Organs Abstracts 4:25, 1975

Hughes DA, Daly BDT, Edmonds CH, Igo SR, Norman JC: An antiarrhythmic regimen for performing bovine cardiac catheterization. Amer Soc Artif Intern Organs Abstracts 3:31, 1974

Hughes DA, Edmonds CH, Igo SR, Daly BDT, Norman JC: External left ventricular performance in the calf during acute ischemia and with abdominal left ventricular assist device (ALVAD) support. Circulation (Supl III) 50(4):167, 1974

Hughes DA, Edmonds CH, Norman JC: An abdominal left ventricular assist device (ALVAD): Patient acceptability survey. Amer Soc Artif Intern Organs Abstracts 3:32, 1974

Hughes DA, Igo SR, Daly BDT, Migliore JJ, Norman JC: Effects of an abdominal left ventricular assist device on myocardial oxygen supply/demand ratios in normally perfused and ischemic bovine myocardium. Ann Thorac Surg 19(3):301, 1975

Hughes DA, Igo SR, Edmonds CH, Migliore JJ, Norman JC: An abdominal left ventricular assist device: Effects on right ventricular output. Proc of 27th Ann Conf on Eng in Med and Biol 16:20, 1974

Igo SR, Carlos CJ, Hibbs CW, Norman JC: Chronic evaluation of cardiac output and left ventricular function during abdominal left ventricular assist device (ALVAD) pumping. Amer Soc Artif Intern Organs Abstracts 4:29, 1975

Igo SR, Edmonds CH, Daly BDT, Hughes DA, Norman JC: Determinants of induced subendocardial ischemia as reflected by DPTI/TTI ratios in occluded and nonoccluded zones of bovine left ventricle. The Physiologist 17(3):253, 1974

Igo SR, Fuqua JM, Edmonds CH, Walker MG, Norman JC: Left ventricular outflow and prosthetic inflow impedances, II: Major factors affecting left ventricular assist device effectiveness. Amer Soc Artif Intern Organs Abstracts 5:38, 1976

Igo SR, Hibbs CW, Fuqua JM, Norman JC: Comparisons of synchronous and asynchronous abdominal left ventricular assist device (ALVAD) pumping. Amer Soc Artif Intern Organs Abstracts 4:29, 1975

Igo SR, Hibbs CW, Fuqua JM, et al: Chronic evaluations of ventricular ejection phase dynamics during abdominal left ventricular assist device (ALVAD) pumping in the awake, unanesthetized calf. Amer Soc for Artif Intern Organs Abstracts 5:38, 1976

Igo SR, Hibbs CW, Fuqua JM, et al: Chronic evaluations of ventricular ejection phase dynamics during abdominal left ventricular assist device (ALVAD) pumping in the awake, unanesthetized calf. Trans Amer Soc Artif Intern Organs 22:480, 1976

Igo SR, Hughes DA, Daly BDT, Huffman FN, Norman JC: Effects of retained blood pump inflow tubes on left ventricular function. Proc of 27th Ann Conf on Eng in Med and Biol 16:125, 1974

Igo SR, Hughes DA, Migliore JJ, Daly BDT, Norman JC: An abdominal left ventricular assist device (ALVAD): Acute and chronic effects on left ventricular mechanics. Abstracts of Coronary Artery Med and Surg Conf. Houston, Texas, Feb. 21–23, 1974, p 126

Igo SR, Hughes DA, Migliore JJ, Daly BDT, Norman JC: An abdominal left ventricular assist device (ALVAD): Acute and chronic effects on left ventricular mechanics. In Norman JC (ed): Coronary Artery Medicine and Surgery: Concepts and Controversies. New York, Appleton, 1975, pp 1006–19

Igo SR, Migliore JJ, Fuqua JM, Norman JC: Effects of an abdominal left ventricular assist device (ALVAD) on myocardial contractility during acute coronary occlusion: Experimental physiologic analyses. J Surg Res 17:177, 1974

Igo SR, Robinson WJ, Hibbs CW, Norman JC: Left ventricular outflow and prosthetic inflow impedances, I: The major determinants of left ventricular assist device effectiveness. Amer Soc for Artif Intern Organs Abstracts 5:38, 1976

Igo SR, Walker MG, Naifeh JG, et al: Effects of transient coronary artery occlusion and left ventricular assist device pumping on diastolic compliance of the bovine left ventricle. Amer Soc Artif Intern Organs Abstracts 5:38, 1976

Liss RH, Edmonds CH, Fuqua JM, Norman JC: Pseudo or neointimal viability: A controversial criteria of artificial heart pump linings. Medical Instrumentation 9(1):81, 1975

Migliore JJ, Arthur J, Fuqua JM, Dove GB, Norman JC: Myocardial arteriovenous oxygen content and derived consumption (qO_2) during abdominal left ventricular assist device (ALVAD) pumping. Clin Res 21(3):438, 1973

Migliore JJ, Dove GB, Fuqua JM, et al: An abdominal left ventricular assist device (ALVAD): Experimental physiologic analyses, IV. Myocardial blood flow. Proc of 26th Ann Conf on Eng in Med and Biol 15:149, 1973

Migliore JJ, Hughes DA, Edmonds CH, et al: An abdominal left ventricular assist device: Resumption of left ventricular pressure generation following profound acute and chronic unloading in the dog and calf. Proc 27th Ann Conf on Eng in Med and Biol 16:121, 1974

Migliore JJ, Robinson WJ, Fuqua JM, et al: An abdominal LVAD: Experimental physiologic analyses, I. Proc 8th Cong of Europ Soc for Exp Surg. Oslo, Norway, May 2–5, 1973

Molokhia FA, Asimacopoulos PJ, Robinson WJ, Huffman FN, Norman JC: Left ventricular assist devices in the calf: Anesthesia, ventilation, antiarrhythmic regimen, and implantation. In Harmison LT (ed): Research Animals in Medicine. DHEW Publication No. (NIH) 72–333, Oct. 2, 1973, pp 383–92

Molokhia FA, Daly BDT, Asimacopoulos PJ, Huffman FN, Norman JC: An antiarrhythmic regimen for left ventricular assist device (LVAD) implantation in the calf. Clin Res 19(4):711, 1971

Naifeh JG, Thompson PA, Johnson MD, et al: Performance of an abdominal left ventricular assist device during induced tachycardias and dysrhythmias. J Thorac Cardiovasc Surg 72(2):1976

Nitta S, Edmonds CH, Carlos CJ, Migliore JJ, Norman JC: Systematic searches for flock emboli in the calf following intracorporeal left ventricular assist device (ALVAD) implantation. Amer Soc Artif Intern Organs Abstracts 4:45, 1975

Norman JC: An abdominal left ventricular assist device (ALVAD): Perspectives and prospects. Cardiovasc Diseases, Bulletin of the Texas Heart Institute 1(3):251, 1974

Norman JC: An intracorporeal (abdominal) left ventricular assist device, 22: Precis and state-of-the-art. Cardiovascular Diseases, Bulletin of the Texas Heart Institute 2(4):425, 1975

Norman JC: Clinical Trials of Left Ventricular Assist Devices. Volume I. Technical Proposal No. 29208-1 for Contract NO1-HL-73-2946, April 15, 1975, p 525

Norman JC, Bernhard WF: Criteria, protocols and reporting forms for initial left ventricular assist device clinical trials (special supplement). Cardiovascular Diseases, Bulletin of the Texas Heart Institute 2(4):438, 1975

Norman JC, Whalen RL, Daly BDT, Migliore JJ, Huffman FN: An implantable abdominal left ventricular assist device (LVAD). Clin Res 20(5):855, 1972

Ponn RB, Scott WC: An abdominal left ventricular assist device: Experimental physiologic analyses. Master's thesis. Harvard University, April 1974

Robinson WJ, Daly BDT, Hughes DA, et al: An abdominal left ventricular assist device: Preclinical studies. Ann Thorac Surg 19(5):540, 1975

Robinson WJ, Igo SR, Daly BDT, et al: An abdominal left ventricular assist device (ALVAD): Chronic hemodynamic analyses in the calf. Amer Soc Artif Intern Organs Abstracts 3:58, 1974

Robinson WJ, Igo SR, Daly BDT, et al: An abdominal left ventricular assist device (ALVAD): Chronic hemodynamic analyses in the calf. Trans Amer Soc Artif Intern Organs 20:709, 1974

Robinson WJ, Maddeaux PR, France NE, Norman JC: Preliminary cost estimates for clinical application of left ventricular assist devices (LVADs). Proc 28th Ann Conf on Eng in Med and Biol 17:359, 1975

Robinson WJ, Migliore JJ, Arthur J, et al: An abdominal left ventricular assist device (ALVAD): Experimental physiologic analyses, II. Trans Amer Soc for Artif Intern Organs 19:229, 1973

Robinson WJ, Molokhia FA, Asimacopoulos PJ, Norman JC: Anesthesia for left ventricular assist device (LVAD) implantation in the calf. Clin Res 19(4):713, 1971

Trono R, Hibbs CW, Fuqua JM, et al: Ex-vivo strength of adherence of neointimas to fibril-flocked surfaces. Amer Soc Artif Intern Organs Abstracts 5:81, 1976

Trono R, Hibbs CW, Fuqua JM, Naifeh JG, Norman JC: Mechanical tensile strength testing of neointimal linings in left ventricular assist devices. Med Instrum 10(1):82, 1976

Walker MG: An abdominal left ventricular assist device (ALVAD): Experimental physiologic analyses. Thesis for Master of Surgery Degree. Aberdeen University (Scotland), 1976

Discussion

MEMBERS OF PANEL

KEITH REEMTSMA, M.D.
Moderator

DAVID BREGMAN, M.D.

ROBERT S. LITWAK, M.D.

JOHN C. NORMAN, M.D.

GEORGE PAPPAS, M.D.

Dr. Reemtsma: There is a question directed to you, Dr. Norman.

What were the plans for these patients following the two to four weeks on the pump? Is it a transplant, and what were your plans?

Dr. Norman: After two to four weeks, we go back and remove the pump in the abdomen, not in the chest.

Dr. Reemtsma: Did you plan new transplants on these patients?

Dr. Norman: No.

Dr. Reemtsma: Dr. Bregman, would you tell us where the EVR equipment is available?

Dr. Bregman: Datascope Corporation, Paramus, New Jersey.

Dr. Reemtsma: Has anyone used the balloon pump secondary to massive pulmonary embolism?

Dr. Pappas: On two occasions, and—well, just temporarily, and the patients died after we took the balloon out.

Dr. Reemtsma: Dr. Litwak, are the cannula fabricated, and are these available commercially?

Dr. Litwak: Yes, they are now made by Hancock Laboratories in Santa Ana, California.

Dr. Reemtsma: Dr. Bregman, what is the balloon in the pulsatile assist device (PAD) made of, and how long has the device been used?

Dr. Bregman: The balloon is made of the same material that the intra-aortic balloon is; it is a fabrication of polyurethane.

The balloon has been used in one procedure for a maximum of about three hours, and we have used it as long as one hour to counterpulsate a patient postoperatively, and that patient survived.

Dr. Reemtsma: We have several questions dealing with the role of anticoagulants.

Each of you can give us a comment on the role of anticoagulants currently used in your cardiac assist devices.

Dr. Litwak: We have been rather hesitant to use simply so-called highly thromboresistant surfaces that are currently available.

Therefore, we have utilized heparin, basically Dr. Hill's protocol, except a little less, running the activated coagulation time (which is normal at about 90 seconds) to about 120 seconds, during higher flows.

Several days later, when we are able to turn the assist pump down, we deliberately increase the heparin to about 180 to 200 seconds, according to the activated clotting time (ACT), and we maintain it at that value until the system is discontinued.

Of the 15 patients, one had to be reexplored because of hemorrhage.

At reexploration, that individual was found to have a bleeding point.

Dr. Pappas: Well, I have had some experience with the other devices. We have used low-dose heparin in patients that have the intra-aortic balloon pump postoperatively, and in some, we did not use heparin at all. We have recently switched over to dextran.

On the partial artificial heart, we use heparin initially and go on to aspirin and Coumadin.

Dr. Bregman: In our preoperative patients, the medical patients, we always anticoagulate with heparin, and in our intraoperative and postoperative patients, the heparin is reversed with Protamine, and aspirin has been used as the sole anticoagulant for the past three years, without incident, to the present time.

There is some evidence to show that the use of dextran may deposit a subcellular particulate background on the balloons (which we had been advised about a few years ago) and we have not been using dextran since these reports came out.

Dr. Reemtsma: Dr. Litwak, do you use a reservoir between the left atrial cannula and the roller pump?

Dr. Litwak: No.

Dr. Reemtsma: There is a question here. What are the prospects for right ventricular unloading?

Who would like to comment on that?

Dr. Norman: It has been done. It is essentially using the same sort of pump as our type of pump on the right side. The longest ones have been done in Boston. They have a right ventricular assist device with the heart fibrillating for about 14 days. This was done in 1968 or 1969, when we met in New Haven.

Dr. Bregman: As far as right ventricular assist devices are concerned, our initial experience has been with right ventricular balloon pumps (a balloon in the cavity of the right ventricle), and we reported this as an abstract, especially when it is used with an intra-aortic balloon, which will offset subendocardial ischemia in the cavity of the right ventricle.

Of course, now, the pulsatile assist device in the intraoperative setting is ideal for us. You can place a cannula in the pulmonary artery and counterpulsate the right heart. It is not too difficult to envision slipping a cannula down the neck and using such a device externally.

Dr. Reemtsma: Dr. Litwak, there is a question for you.

Are there any long-term problems with embolic phenomena in your device?

Dr. Litwak: We have not had any clinical evidence in the individuals dismissed from the hospital, and insofar as clinical evidence of emboli in the hospital, we have not seen evidence of that as well.

I think it would be naive of us to think that there are not small microemboli; but the problem is that we don't yet have adequate methods of assessing what is going on during the left heart pumping. Clearly, this is something that needs to be looked at, but from a clinical standpoint, we have not seen a problem.

Dr. Reemtsma: Dr. Bregman, what modifications are required in either the aortic cannulation or the arterial line for PAD use?

Would you comment on this?

Dr. Bregman: Yes, the beauty of this device is in its simplicity and its nondisturbance of the cardiac surgeon. The usual aortic cannula is used, and it probably can be used with smaller cannulae as well, since we have experience with one pediatric patient with good pulsation.

The device is in the operating field, usually to the side of the first assistant, and it is out of the way. Once the procedure begins, the surgeon does not even know it is being used.

Dr. Reemtsma: Dr. Norman, how do you define DPTI and TTI with your system?

Dr. Norman: It is summed up in the article of the Annals of Thoracic Surgery, the date of 1974, beginning of 1975, and it requires some mathematical manipulation, but in essence the slide that Dr. Bregman showed you with the balloon pump on and off demonstrated this nicely.

We get the same thing, only about eight to ten times more effectively. It is in the Bibliography of my chapter.

Dr. Reemtsma: Dr. Norman, there is another question that is directed to you regarding the changes in the inflow and outflow connectors with the device you discussed today. The question is, were these changes made in response to changes in the human anatomy of these patients, or for other reasons?

Dr. Norman: No, the changes were made in response to experimental preparations. I did not go into these details, but prior to our initial clinical trials, there were human studies in cadavers. These were prerequisites that were set down by federal auspices, among a number of other constraints.

Dr. Reemtsma: What method of sterilization is used in the preparation of that device, or do they come in a nonsterile state?

Dr. Norman: We send them down to Houston International. We sterilize them on receipt in our laboratories. We have kept them sterile. But the biomaterial starts to degrade once you initiate sterilization. We feel now in the type of logistics we have worked out (and this is in our next report) that there is no reason to keep one sterile. There is adequate time for it to be sterilized before it is used, once you have identified the patient.

Dr. Reemtsma: Dr. Pappas, the effect of pulsatile blood flow on organs other than the heart and how these are affected by the system that you use is the next question.

I know that you have had considerable interest in that. Could you bring us up to date on your thoughts on this subject?

Dr. Pappas: Well, first of all, we have seen very little evidence of renal failure afterward, in contrast to other patients who were operated on with nonpulsatile flow.

We determined that LDH levels were better in the pulsatile flow, indicating better tissue perfusion.

We also found lower levels of SGOT postoperatively, which may indicate less cellular injury.

Dr. Reemtsma: Do you have a controlled series of patients who do not receive the pulsatile assist device?

Dr. Bregman: Yes, we have concurrent controls, and of

course, we have our entire clinical series before we began pulsating. The urine data I reported happened to be with the same patients done at the same time without pulsation, so that it was an equally matched series.

In fact, the patients pulsated in general, were sicker, so that the responses were certainly comparable, as were the other data.

Dr. Reemtsma: Another question is antibiotic coverage in these patients.

Would you start, Dr. Litwak?

Dr. Litwak: I think some of the classic studies initially done at Massachusetts General clearly indicate that in patients undergoing body perfusion, a preventive and antibacterial action is mandated, and therefore, we maintain it throughout the circulatory system, starting, of course, preoperatively with the conventional administration of antibiotics.

The only special managements that we employ are at the two exit points of the extracorporeal tubing, where we put some ointment. Other than that, we do nothing else but administer conventional antibiotics.

Dr. Pappas: We do it postoperatively.

Dr. Norman: Our patients are run essentially the way all patients are. I think there are no changes in their routine management, which involves antibiotics.

We did not have an incidence of sepsis. I think that the longest one I have done was in Boston (before going down to Houston)—and was about 27 days—and it was not a big problem.

Dr. Bregman: We employ antibiotics routinely in the balloon patients beginning with the insertion of the balloon.

Our open heart protocol calls for five days of antibiotics postoperatively.

We feel that while the balloon is in place, since there is a vascular prosthesis that is exposed to the outside, in essence, by the balloon catheter, it is wise to use antibiotic coverage. With this regimen, we have not had a wound infection to the present time.

Dr. Reemtsma: There is a question that I will read and ask you to comment on.

There have been some strong comments on the importance of pulsatile versus nonpulsatile cardiopulmonary bypass.

Are there any comments on the physiologic acceptability of nonpulsatile assist in long-term ventricular assist cases? Dr. Norman?

Dr. Norman: The classic reference on pulsatile perfusion was published in the medical journals of the Royal Academy of Medicine in about 1900. If you are interested in the review of it, you can refer to it.

Cardio-pulmonary bypass is a controlled form of shock, and if you can pulsate your flow for the duration of cardiopulmonary bypass, you will have a better perfusion.

Nonpulsatile is adequate. Pulsatile is probably better.

Dr. Pappas: Well, I certainly agree. There are many reports about the effectiveness of pulsatile flow in the literature, and the big question I have is what if we take an individual and pump him with a nonpulsatile flow, will he awaken? How long will it last? That is something that needs to be answered.

Dr. Litwak: Well, I am certainly convinced that man has had a fairly long run with pulsatile flow, and the evidence is clear that it works.

But then, of course, when you are applying biological engineering problems, there is always a cost/benefit ratio. The data remain unclear, primarily because our methodology is inadequate to clearly assess the questions that have to be answered.

Therefore, intuitively, we all agree that pulsatile flow is the thing to achieve. The evidence is really not defensible in terms of hard science, but the point is that there is a suggestion that the experimental animal *man* was right, and the engineer upstairs who designed it knew what he was doing.

Dr. Norman: I think it is a bit of a travesty to discuss this with Dr. Galletti in the front row.

Dr. Bregman: I just wanted to make a point that has not come up so far.

Dr. Habal of our laboratory, and others have done some nice studies showing how pulsatile flow is especially beneficial in the fibrillating heart, and I think that it is another advantage of the whole process.

Dr. Reemtsma: There is a question here addressed to Dr. Norman and Dr. Litwak and it asks the comparative virtues of the two types of blood ventricular assist devices and refers to the need of complicated reoperation. I think that the implication is, how do you balance out the reoperation in the two devices that Dr. Litwak and Dr. Norman are discussing?

Dr. Litwak: I think it is hard to know at this stage. I think from a physiologic standpoint, based on what we know about the physiologic aspects of myocardial recovery, if one worships at the altar of oxygen consumption as a criteria to be achieved above all else, there is no question that total unloading of the left ventricle is the thing to do. But recognize that the patients in the hospital who have the lowest MVO_2's are in the autopsy room.

It may very well be that we are worshipping at the altar of the wrong god.

Please don't misunderstand. I can see that thermodynamic laws are immutable, and nothing I am saying convinces me that things have changed during the millions of years where they have seemed to do pretty well.

However, the question, the key question, is what criteria do we have for defining myocardial recovery? And the answer is, we really don't know yet. So the point is that from our standpoint, I have to go back to some intuitive questions. One, does the partial left heart assist device seem to stabilize the patient's metabolic and hemodynamic rates? Secondly, are patients who have been unable to be weaned off by conventional bypass able to achieve myocardial recovery? The answer is yes.

In point of fact, the simplicity of the method based upon our clinical evidence (and that is all we have), plus indirect measurements, suggest that from what we know, the system seems to work.

I am not suggesting it is the greatest thing since sliced bread, I am only saying right now, in view of our limited knowledge, it seems to work.

Dr. Reemtsma: Dr. Norman, do you want to comment?

Dr. Norman: Yes, I agree with everything that has been said and I particularly agree with Dr. Litwak.

I would like to point out that were it not for Dr. Litwak, we would not be underway, because he is chairman of one of the committees in Washington, and his system is a good system.

We think our system will be a longer-lived system. We think our system will develop into a permanent implant.

Dr. Reemtsma: Where does the total artificial heart fit in now, Dr. Norman?

Could you wrap that one up for us, so to speak?

Dr. Norman: It is a difficult question. I am not sure how I feel about total artificial hearts. I am certain that the research should be done. It is a complex problem. It took us six years to come to these initial creeping steps of partial left ventricle assist devices.

I think that they can be depended upon. I think there are many problems. The longest survivor, I think, is somewhere in the range of about four months.

I have just seen in Houston total artificial hearts fabricated in Russia and flown to the Methodist Hospital with pulsatile atria and ventricles. It is a research area that is well worthwhile.

There is a certain aura and mystique about artificial hearts which they don't deserve. They are blood pumps fabricated and tested to be compatible. I think the future in this area is great. It is beset with problems, but we are making progress.

Dr. Reemtsma: Thank you for the last question, and I would like to ask each of the panelists to answer this.

The question is, are any of these devices cost-effective, and I think you understand the implications of this. But perhaps we might ask each of you to comment on the cost of what each of us is talking about, and I don't mean just dollars, but staffing. What demands are made of our nurses, hospital staff, intensive care units and so forth?

I know that this is a big order, but I think that this is something that would be of interest.

Dr. Litwak: This is a very important question, and a major undertaking in terms of the assignment of personnel, production of personnel, technical staff, and data acquisition.

We calculate that one patient placed on the left heart assist system probably costs in the order of $25,000 in terms of supportive management, additional personnel, and so on.

Dr. Pappas: Well, I haven't had any experience with long-term support. I think that perhaps pulsatile flow will reduce the cost by preserving the myocardium.

Dr. Norman: We have been fortunate because we have been able to shape our situation in Houston based on the mistakes we made in other places. Our balloon pump system is centralized, and it is all computerized. We can essentially say that it adds about $300 or $400 a day to a patient's bill.

Open heart surgery costs somewhere between $5000 and $6000 in Houston, in an uncomplicated case. If we get any difficulties, it can double.

With regard to the left ventricular assist device cost effectiveness, there is a proposal that is referenced in my chapter, which is about 525 pages in length. We analyzed the costs of all our patients for a year. We estimated that it will increase the cost to a patient about 25 percent above that of the intra-aortic balloon pump.

Now, we are working with prototypes, and it requires a highly trained staff.

We are totally dedicated to it. What we are doing is exploring areas that have not been explored. People like to know how much does this cost?

The console, which is a prototype (there are two), costs somewhere in the range of $40,000. They can be made for a tenth of that.

I think that there are people who can sell you a ventricular assist device, and the cost is somewhere between $3,000 and $4,000. I just throw that out as information. I am not associated with that group of people.

I think the amount of money that is spent on the program is miniscule in terms of the potential that the program has in saving lives.

Balloons were gadgets 10 years ago, and people like Dr. Bregman, who were still in junior high school then, were working on them.

Now, there are 5000 patients who have undergone intra-aortic balloon pumping. These figures are increasing, and it is spreading into the community hospital. It is a tremendous contribution, but someone had to fight for it 10 years ago, to make it readily available. We are giving seminars on intra-aortic balloon pumps for people in Galveston and over in Port Rio and Louisiana.

This is not that big a deal, and you can tell one of the nurses to leave and set up a unit somewhere else.

Our resident is set up, and he will be doing them in July. It is pretty straightforward.

Dr. Reemtsma: Dr. Bregman, could you bring us up to date on your views of the cost-effectiveness and also staffing that would be necessary for the function of an intra-aortic balloon pump system in an institution such as this, and in particular, the changing patterns with increasing experience in institutions.

Dr. Bregman: I think the last statement is the key, because with any of these new techniques, in the beginning, the technique naturally requires more supportive people and a very highly organized team.

At the present time, for example, in the Presbyterian Hospital, we have two individuals who know how to run the machinery quite well. They always stand by when a balloon is inserted and tune up the machine, and then the house staff performs any further manipulations of the equipment, since little manipulation is needed.

Presently, the residents insert all of the balloons. So, in fact, what it costs in this hospital anyway, would be the cost of the balloon, which is about $250, the depreciation of the equipment, and part of the salaries of the individuals, and I suppose it would come to about $300 or $400 a day.

As far as the PAD is concerned, the cost of these disposable items is less than the balloon. I agree with Dr. Pappas, because I think that since we are preserving the myocardium better, we will use fewer balloons and the cost-effectiveness will probably be much greater. In addition, the total hospitalization may be shorter with a reduction in both morbidity and mortality.

Dr. Reemtsma: We are pleased to have a distinguished representative from Dr. Valeriy Shumakov's group in Moscow with us today.

Professor Ergorov: I am the Chief of the Artificial Heart Laboratories at the Institute of Transplantation of Organs and Tissues, Ministry of Public Health, USSR. Later this month, with my colleagues, we are going to participate in the joint implantation of the artificial heart with the United States.

I would like to thank Dr. Bregman and Dr. Reemtsma for this opportunity to participate in the symposium.

In our clinic and in the Clinic of Experimental Surgery, we are using methods of mechanical circulatory assistance and other methods.

Since the time is limited, I would just like to say a few words on the mechanical circulatory assist devices.

Four years ago, Dr. Bregman visited our country and shared with us his experience which was at that point just in the beginning stages. The method of using the balloon pump has subsequently been used on 96 patients in our country. The first group of patients in whom we applied the balloon pump method were patients with cardiogenic shock.

Since we had difficulties with coordinating the internists and the surgeons and other personnel, we also carefully chose our patients.

The criteria were as follows: Arterial pressure less than 80 mm Hg (the hypertensive patient is up to 100 mm Hg), oliguria, pulmonary capillary wedge pressure up to 20 or 25 mm Hg. About 15 percent of patients survived from this group.

The second group of patients in which we used the balloon were patients with preinfarction angina. We did not have any difficulties with this group. They were observed during a period of one year. The balloon pump was also applied to patients after heart surgery, and the results are not well known yet. However, we are very hopeful.

At the present time, we are working on the method of external counterpulsation.

We have a few methods of applying this. Going back a bit in history, the patient wears a suit. The suit is the same model used on the cosmonauts. In the last method of external counterpulsation, bands are used and can be moved from place to place when necessary.

This method is highly advantageous. First, it is very useful and logical as well because you can apply it very fast. You can also use it in ambulances; we have applied it a few times in ambulances while the patient was being transported to the clinic.

There is another functional advantage of this system. We have other arterial methods, but using this method, we can apply it to the venous system as well. This method is also used internally. It is now in experimental stages. The results are very good. Thank you for your attention.

Dr. Bregman: Thank you Dr. Ergorov for sharing with us the current status of mechanical circulatory assistance in the Soviet Union.

Dr. Reemtsma: Thank you. This concludes the morning session.

I would like to thank the panelists and in particular, I would like to thank the audience.

CHAPTER 5

Background and Technical Aspects of Membrane Oxygenation

Pierre M. Galletti

Membrane oxygenation was first devised as a tool for cardiac surgery. The earliest experience with membrane lungs demonstrated that however imperfect and cumbersome such devices were at the time, they nonetheless produced less damage during extracorporeal blood handling than the conventional oxygenators, and could provide several hours of continuous service without apparent loss in effectiveness. Thus quite naturally, investigators thought of using extracorporeal membrane oxygenation (ECMO, as it came to be named) to achieve extended respiratory support in potentially reversible lung disease. The purpose of this chapter is to review the background and the technology of membrane oxygenation, the obstacles it has faced during its development, and eventually, to philosophize as to where it may be going.

HISTORIC BACKGROUND

As in the case with almost any application of biotechnology, membrane oxygenation started with casual, but nevertheless astute observations by pioneers endowed with vision and perseverance (Table 1). As is also often the case, the very first phase of development extended all the way to clinical application, in spite of what appears in retrospect a limited understanding of the controlling processes, formidable technical difficulties, and a surprising lack of recognition among peers for the ultimate potential of the newly proposed approach.

TABLE 1. Clinical Observations and Fundamental Concepts

	YEAR	
Oxygenation of venous blood through dialysis	1944	Kolff
Evaluation of cellulosic membrane oxygenator	1951	Karlson
Large scale, sandwich type of membrane oxygenator	1955	Clowes
Clinical validation in open heart surgery	1957	Clowes
Reinforced (coated fabric) silicone resin membrane	1958	Thomas
CO_2 bottleneck with Teflon membranes	1958	Melrose, Peirce
Silicone rubber membranes	1960	Dow-Corning
Oxygen transport limitation by fluid films	1960	Peirce, Marx
Microporous membrane materials	1960	McCaughan

In fact, the concept of membrane oxygenation started with the clinical observation that during the course of hemodialysis using the rotating-drum kidney, venous blood channeled through cellophane tubing would turn red upon prolonged exposure to an aerated dialysis medium. Investigators soon realized that gas exchange between watery media separated by a hydrophilic membrane had to be quite inefficient because of the diffusion distances involved. Furthermore, it would present many other problems, such as acid-base balance, electrolyte and solute exchange, control of ultrafiltration, etc. Thus, the search turned toward relatively hydrophobic plastics: Polyethylene and ethylcellulose were first tried without much success because they proved to be quite impermeable to gases. In the mid-fifties, however, Teflon became available in the form of thin sheets or membrane rolls which proved reliably pinhole-free because of the quality control required in the industrial application (capacitors) for which this material was produced. This permitted a major advance on the part of G.H.A. Clowes, who designed in Cleveland the first operational clinical membrane oxygenator. At about the same time in Paris, J.A. Thomas fabricated a microporous membrane by coating a silicone over a textile mesh stretched over a rotating drum. The design of the original Clowes and Thomas membrane oxygenators were successfully applied in over 100 clinical perfusions for open heart surgery, a tribute to the creativity and perseverence of cardiovascular surgeons. However, the equipment was cumbersome and the cost such that it could not realistically compete with the sturdy, reliable bubble or disc oxygenators that were just then coming into favor.

This set of circumstances led, throughout the sixties, to a long period of incubation of membrane lung technology. Important conceptual and experimental advances were made, without, however, reaching a stage of practicality that would permit the membrane oxygenator to compete with the standard surgical instruments, that eventually evolved into sleek, see-through, disposable devices. The milestones of membrane oxygenator development during that decade are listed in Table 2. They include fundamen-

TABLE 2. Period of Transition

	YEAR	
Logistics of multiple-layer, parallel-flow devices	1961	Peirce
Multiple-point support for flat membrane sheets	1961	Galletti, Peirce
Pressurized "shim" to stabilize blood flow distribution	1962	Harvey
Combined artificial lung-kidney machine (Klung)	1962	Hopf, Galletti
Screen-in-blood concept of bloodstream mixing	1965	Bramson
Concept of an implantable lung	1965	Bodell
Pattern definition on membrane surfaces	1966	Peirce
Ultrathin silicone rubber membrane	1966	Burns, Melrose
Silicone-polycarbonate copolymer	1966	General Electric

tal observations and ingenious design ideas promoted by a coterie of tenacious investigators who anticipated most of the practical advances that were to florish in the seventies.

The recognition around 1958–59 of the favorable gas permeability properties of silicone polymers, coupled with technological advances that permitted manufacturing this material in the form of thin sheets, were the key elements in further progress of membrane oxygenation. Now investigators could compare not only various thicknesses of the same Teflon membrane, but also another material with quite different transport properties. Even before permeability had been measured in recognizable standard units, E.C. Peirce and T.I. Marx had independently made the fundamental observation that given membrane materials with permeability properties equal to, or better than, those of silicone rubber and Teflon, the oxygen transfer capacity of a membrane lung would not be limited by the nature of the plastic membrane itself, but by the thickness of the blood boundary layer adjacent to it. Hence the generalization that dominated membrane lung design until recently: CO_2 transfer is limited by the chemical nature and the thickness of the polymer membrane, but O_2 transfer is primarily controlled by the geometry of the blood path.

This view encouraged developmental work not solely toward thinner membranes (typically obtained by coating a silicone polymer suspension over a textile cloth), but also toward uneven membrane surfaces, which could be expected to induce some degree of convective mixing in the blood layer immediately adjacent to the membrane. The word "turbulence" was often used to describe the desired blood mixing, much to the dismay of engineers who could not recognize in these early prototypes well-defined flow geometrics authorizing the use of precise fluid dynamics concepts. Nevertheless, improvements in blood oxygenation could demonstrably be obtained by proper selection of the mesh size and fiber orientation in textile-reinforced membranes, by using knit rather than single-strand fabrics, by embossing or engraving a particular pattern on the membrane sheet itself, or by the simple expedient of sandwiching a wide-mesh screen within the blood layer between adjacent plastic membranes. This last design concept, employed on a large scale in the 5.6-meter^2 Bramson-Gerbode oxygenator, led to the second wave of clinical application in the mid-sixties, furthering once more surgical interest in this category of devices.

The dilemma of membrane lung design became increasingly clear as membrane materials could be experimentally characterized for their permeability properties, and design problems could be expressed in terms of mass transfer theory derived from chemical engineering. As the influence of blood flow pattern and blood flow distribution began to be quantitatively analyzed, a step forward in performance and reliability could be observed, recruiting a new group of believers in the future of membrane oxygenation.

Better flow designs led to a renewed demand for improved membranes, and stimulated three major technical advances: the synthesis and fabrication of the General Electric polycarbonate-silicone copolymer, which could be made into thinner sheets than the parent silicone because of the mechanical strength imparted by the polycarbonate; the unraveling (in a London hospital) of a new technology for the fabrication of ultrathin, pinhole-free, unsupported silicone rubber membranes; and finally, the industrial production (Dow Chemical) of very small, very thin-walled tubes of silicone copolymer, known in the trade as hollow fibers. Hollow fibers, assembled in a bundle and potted together at both ends with silicone elastomers, epoxys or polyurethanes, struck the clinician's imagination because their parallel arrangement so closely resembled our intuitive image of a capillary bed. For a while, it seemed that the hollow-fiber approach would be the ultimate answer to membrane lung design, until recurring problems of thrombus formation on the "face sheet" of the fiber bundle identified the Achilles' heel of such devices. Because hollow fibers claimed an ancestry in textile technology, it was not long before someone thought of weaving them as a cloth, and to design a filter-pack type of oxygenator, with the gas circulating through the lumen of the fibers and blood in the interstices between them, in short, a reversed capillary bed.

Parallel with these technological advances, the seeds were planted for new concepts in artificial organs. The Klung design demonstrated that blood-gas exchange and hemodialysis could be combined in a single artificial lung-kidney in which the blood was simultaneously exposed to two types of membrane for two different exchange processes. Surgical imagination led to the very first prototype for an implantable artificial lung, based on parallel bundles of thin-walled silicone rubber tubing inserted in Teflon envelopes within the chest. The original booster lung, limited as it was by the shortcomings of available "biomaterials," could only provide limited and temporary support. Nonetheless, it expanded the horizons of membrane oxygenation in directions which will be felt for decades.

The late 1960s and the early 1970s witnessed the encounter of science, technology, and industry (Table 3). Biomaterials science finally emerged as a respectable academic endeavor and attracted a group of distinguished physical scientists who started making some order of what had been heretofore empirical knowledge. The biocompatibility of polymers was systematically investigated. Advances in plastic technology were applied to fabrication problems such as casting, molding, gluing, and sealing of membrane oxygenator parts, leading to great simplification in design and assembly of newer prototypes. Industry became involved, and with the commercialization of the Lande-Edwards oxygenator, problems of large scale production, reliability, quality control, sterilization, shelf-life, and shipping were for the first time confronted and resolved. The distribution of that standardized, ready to use, disposable membrane oxygenator did much to broaden the ranks of those who could promote the field in the laboratory or in the clinic.

TABLE 3. Beginning of Industrial Era

	YEAR	
Industrial development of a disposable oxygenator	1965	Lande-Edwards
Physical characterization of membrane permeability	1966	Galletti, Snider
Liquid-liquid (fluorocarbon) oxygenators	1968	Clark
Gas-permeable hollow fibers	1969	Dow Chemical
Hydrophobic microporous membrane materials	1969	Dantowitz, Lautier
NIH Medical Device Application Program	1970	Hastings, Dennis

Over a period of about five years, the Artificial Heart Program of the National Institutes of Health made a significant investment in membrane oxygenation. This included the fabrication of new polymers, the development of new designs, and attempts with new exchange processes. For a while, there seemed to be a dozen competing approaches that all had a reasonable chance of culminating in clinically useful devices. Ironically, the models that have survived the evolutionary process and reached the commercial production stage trace their origin in industrial rather than in government support. However, one should not underestimate the leavening influence of a national program of oxygenator fabrication and evaluation. Frequent meetings among investigators led to a greater degree of standardization in reporting oxygenator performance data, and in time, to a more general consensus about the advantages and drawbacks of membrane oxygenation. Through that effort, oxygenator modules reached such a level of performance and reliability that they could seriously be considered for total body perfusion as required in cardiac surgery.

Four main lines of research have dominated the membrane lung field since 1970 (Table 4). Some investigators have attempted to revive the concept of liquid-to-liquid exchangers through sophisticated designs utilizing liquids of high oxygen-carrying capacity. Others have pursued various fluid dynamic approaches to minimize the obstacle to oxygen transport resulting from the fluid boundary layer adjacent to the exchange membrane. Still others have violated the taboo against direct blood-gas interface and successfully experimented with microporous membranes. Finally, a last group has concentrated its efforts toward the elimination of membrane surface imperfections thought to be responsible for platelet deposition and eventually thrombosis in the extracorporeal circuit.

TABLE 4. Encounter of Science, Technology, and Industry

	YEAR	
Clinical, long-term respiratory support	1970	Hill
Progress with the spiral-coil membrane oxygenator	1970	Kolobow, Zapol
Standardization of gas transfer performance analysis	1972	Galletti, Richardson
Secondary flows generated by external forces	1972	Drinker, Bartlett, Melrose
Secondary flows inherent to blood flow path geometry	1972	Mockross, Dorson
Secondary flows associated with blood pulsation	1973	Bellhouse

Liquid-liquid exchangers are still in the experimental stage. For a while, the accent was placed on liquid fluorocarbons, which are transparent organic liquids with a very high coefficient of solubility for oxygen and carbon dioxide. These liquids are immiscible with water or blood, and because of their high specific gravity, can be made to flow in direct contact with blood without mixing, the interface between the two liquids acting as a virtual membrane across which oxygen and carbon dioxide can be traded from one fluid to the other. Elegant designs have been proposed to accomplish this in a continuous manner, and the efficiency of the process has been well established. Two factors, however, have discouraged clinical application: the mechanical complexity of the systems (which must be backed by a bubble oxygenator to load the flurocarbon with oxygen and remove its carbon dioxide), and the danger of fluorocarbon embolism into the bloodstream. The pharmacology and toxicology of these complex organic liquids is far from being elucidated, and thus liquid fluorcarbon oxygenators have remained heretofore a laboratory curiosity.

An equally intriguing approach is that of blood exchange via hemodialysis through catalytic membranes. Here the concept is to expose blood to water soluble precursors or derivatives of the respiratory gases. This means, in practice, hemodialysis against a liquid containing a large source of oxygen (hydrogen peroxide solution) and a sink for carbon dioxide (chemical binding of bicarbonate with a strong base). A transition metal oxide (ruthenium oxide has been found to be the most effective) is deposited within the mesh of cellulosic membranes otherwise similar to those used in hemodialysis. The catalyst is fixed and does not leach out into the blood or the hydrogen peroxide solution. A chemical reaction occurs within the fluid-filled cellulosic matrix, and oxygen is liberated in immediate contact with the blood that flows adjacent to the membrane. The effectiveness of this system has been well established with laboratory prototypes. However, two main difficulties remain: One is the leakage into the blood of minute quantities of hydrogen peroxide, which at least in a catalase-poor animal such as the dog, leads to progressive methemoglobinemia. The other problem is that ultimate binding of carbon dioxide in the form of carbonates, also leads to a loss of calcium, magnesium, and phosphates, which must then be compensated by intravenous infusion of appropriate salt solutions to the perfused subject.

A number of approaches have been proposed to control and minimize the blood boundary layer that effectively limits oxygen transport in laminar flow systems. They all rely on the promotion of convective transport within the blood phase in order to mix and homogenize the blood as it flows through the exchange device. The term "secondary flow" is used by fluid dynamicists to designate convective transport within a moving fluid at an angle or in a plane different from that of the main throughflow. Such mechanisms have been empirically used since the beginning of membrane oxygenation, but it is only in recent years that detailed engineering analysis has led to artificial lung configurations that take maximum advantage of these phenomena.

It would not be possible here to review all systems that have been proposed. The oscillating toroidal chamber of P.A. Drinker and R.H. Bartlett, the grooved plate and highly pulsatile flow of the Oxford-Bellhouse oxygenator, and the rotating microporous disc-membrane oxygenator of J.D. Hill, are the best known of these systems. All have demonstrated a remarkable gas transport efficiency in laboratory prototypes, and the latter at least has been successfully employed in cardiac surgery. Nevertheless, many surgeons find these oxygenators still mechanically too complex and delicate to be used without afterthought in the operating room.

The concept of using microporous materials to eliminate the membrane resistance factor in gas transport between oxygen and blood was promulgated simultaneously in the United States and in France around 1969. Against the conventional wisdom of the time, experimentalists on both sides of the Atlantic surmised that through a microporous hydrophobic material, oxygen and blood could be brought into direct contact without actually mixing because surface tension would keep both phases separated. Prototypes demonstrated the feasibility of such systems, and also their remarkable gas exchange efficiency. Then followed a phase of industrial research and development which took advantage of the relatively low cost of microporous materials (initially Teflon in the United States, silicone-coated paper in France). The net result has been the design and distribution at a competitive price of compact, disposable membrane lungs fully capable of meeting the needs of cardiac surgery. Efforts continue to identify the ideal porosity of membrane materials, the precise nature of the blood-material interface in gas-filled polymers, and the potential advantages of lining microporous substrates with ultrathin coats of a nonporous substance.

The last area of development in recent years has been the recognition that surface irregularities such as protruding silica crystals on the exposed surface of silicone rubber membranes are indeed responsible to a major extent for platelet deposition on blood-exposed membranes. Such membrane irregularities have been incriminated in the development of thromboembolic phenomena in the extracorporeal circuit. Conversely, membranes prepared in a manner to minimize this problem, such as silica-free silicone rubber, have been shown to allow perfusion with minimal doses of anticoagulants. Several membrane materials are currently under investigation from the standpoint of improved platelet compatibility without losing the necessary permeability to oxygen and carbon dioxide. Carbon may eventually replace silica as the filler in silicone elastomers. Ethylcellulose perfluorobutyrate and polyalkylsulfones seem to be at the present time at the forefront of competitors with the more traditional membrane materials. Progress in material formulation, the use of clean room fabrication and assembly techniques in the manufacturing of membrane lungs, and a better appreciation of the membrane-blood interactions have probably all played a role in the success reported by several investigators with the use of minimal doses of heparin. It is now possible to utilize extracorporeal membrane oxygenation for several days, indeed several weeks, with heparin dosages at least one order of magnitude below those customarily employed in surgical perfusions.

TECHNICAL ASSESSMENT

From this survey of membrane lung history, and the concurrent experience in parallel fields of biotechnology (prosthetic valves, artificial hearts, hemodialysis equipment, etc.), some conclusions can be derived which should help us to appreciate where we stand at the present time, and in which direction progress may be made.

Modern membrane lungs are effective inasmuch as they can easily cover the gas exchange needs of a normothermic adult. Since anesthetized, hemodiluted, moderately hypothermic patients under perfusion have a reduced metabolism, current membrane lungs, without necessarily reaching the peak performance of an efficient bubble oxygenator, do nevertheless provide enough of a safety margin for the perfusionist to feel secure under any clinical situation. Possibly the most important aspect of effectiveness of membrane lungs is their unflinching performance regardless of the duration of perfusion. Properly employed, and certainly within the most generous time boundaries of present-day cardiac surgery, membrane lungs display a constant performance. When used for long-term respiratory support, membrane oxygenators are no longer the bottleneck. Some investigators have adopted a routine of changing the oxygenator module at three- to five-day intervals, primarily to minimize the risk of thrombus formation and subsequent embolism when minimal doses of heparin are used. The gas transfer capacity remains remarkably stable, and there is usually no performance decay to compound the biological problems of unexpectedly long perfusion.

Membrane lungs are said to be safe, meaning that the trauma imposed on blood by continuing recirculation outside of the body is less than that observed with the more traditional bubbling or filming systems. The scientific evidence for this is well established for long-term respiratory assistance, but is not entirely unequivocal for surgical perfusions. The ambiguity stems in part from the fact that the design of coronary suction systems, and the manner in which such systems are used in the operating room, are much more important as potential sources of blood trauma than the blood oxygenator itself. Thus, changing the gas exchange device alone is not a recipe for trouble-free postperfusion periods. Nevertheless, several surgeons have reported an easier blood pressure control, less postoperative confusion, and earlier awakening and recovery in patients perfused with membrane oxygenators, compared with conventional equipment.

Membrane lungs are reliable because they are geometrically much better defined than their competitors of the bubble or disc type. The blood compartment of a membrane lung is closed to atmospheric pressure, and its content is almost constant (excluding fluctuations associated with the compliance of the membranes). This provides a measure of protection against unrecognized change in circulating blood volume, which is of particular value in long-term respiratory support. In surgical perfusions, however, this may be a mixed blessing. On the one side, a fixed blood volume in the extracorporeal circuit eliminates ambiguities in the patient blood pressure and volume control associated with fluctuations in blood level of the oxygenator. On the other hand, it is not possible to conduct a surgical perfusion without a blood reserve in the circuit, and thus distensible reservoirs must be included for safety sake. Because the blood volume in the oxygenator is fixed, blood flow in and out of the device must be accurately matched, otherwise the gas exchange unit would collapse or explode. Blood circuits and pumping mechanisms must include safety features to prevent such accidents. In some designs of membrane lungs, the problem cannot be visually anticipated in as direct a manner as through the change in blood level in a disposable bubble oxygenator, and the perfusion team must have other warning systems at hand. The availability of input-controlled blood pumps, whether in the form of servo-control from a collapsible "atrium" (T. Kolobow, W.M. Zapol) or by virtue of the geometric design of the pumping chambers (Rhone-Poulenc), has done much to improve the practicality of extracorporeal membrane oxygenation.

The last characteristic of the modern membrane lung is to be a disposable, moderate-cost item. Because membrane lungs rely on narrow, geometrically well-defined blood paths, arranged in a complex manner within a sealed box, it is practically impossible to clean them after use to a point where they could be reused clinically. This brings into consideration the issue of cost. One of the most positive results of the increasing competition among membrane lung manufacturers for the cardiac surgery market is the progressive lowering of prices. This is associated in part with volume of production, labor-saving assembly techniques, and in recent years, the advent of new membrane materials inherently less expensive than the classic silicone polymers of Teflons. On the world market, there are currently five or six types of membrane lungs that have successfully been used in perfusions lasting several days.

REMAINING PROBLEM AREAS

With the increasing acceptance of membrane lungs for cardiac surgery or long-term respiratory assistance, and the technical progress associated with keen competition between manufacturers, the field of membrane oxygenation could well be considered as provisionally settled. New major challenges, however, seem to fascinate investigators and are likely to occupy their attention in the years to come. One such challenge relates to the regulation of gas transfer in the extracorporeal device.

The performance of any membrane lung is blood flow and gas flow dependent, and varies in accordance with fluctuations of controlling parameters (eg, oxygen saturation, pCO_2) in the blood drained from the patient. Autoregulation of this system has not yet developed as a clinical priority, largely because the patient's respiratory reflexes and his remaining lung exchange capacity have provided the necessary adjustments. There may come a time, however, for increased sophistication if biologic difficulties can be associated with the relative "insensitivity" of present-day devices.

In terms of membrane lung design, it is all too clear that we need better mainfolding and branching systems in the blood circuit. Artificial organs, unlike their natural counterparts, are built of assembled components and not in continuity. Detailed observations of membrane lungs after clinical use shows that thrombogenic problems often arise at the transition between components. New technologies are needed to build branching blood channels in continuity with the feeder structure, and there is still a long way to go before this can be accomplished with the elegance and energy conservation of our vascular system.

One obvious aspect of the difference in evolutionary maturity between natural and artificial lung is illustrated by the low pressure head required from the right ventricle, as compared to the propulsion component of a pump-oxygenator. As membrane lungs reach a stage of efficiency which allow us to entertain the dream of an implantable "booster lung," more consideration will have to be given to low-resistance exchange devices and their adaptation as lung prostheses.

Very much with us is the problem of connecting an extracorporeal membrane oxygenator to the vascular system. Stated candidly, much less effort has been expended by manufacturers on arterial and venous catheters than on oxygenators and pumps. The result is that vascular connections are often the mechanical weak point of the system, and occasionally limit the value of the biological assistance provided by the mechanical system. Well-directed progress in catheter technology should eventually offset this difficulty.

OUTLOOK FOR THE FUTURE

Looking forward to the next few years of progress, several lines of research seem to warrant investigation (Table 5). One such field is the tailoring of microporous membranes toward the specific function of gas exchange. Much remains unexplained as to the exact physical nature of blood-gas interaction at the microporous interface. The possibility of membrane polarization, the value of specific chemicals, the detailed formulation of microporous polymer and their lining with live cells or hemocompatible materials may well lead to new modalities of application of microporous membrane devices.

TABLE 5. Outlook

	YEAR	
Enhancement of gas transport through catalytic membranes	1972	Updyke
Clinical microporous membrane oxygenator	1973	Murphy
Rotating microporous membrane oxygenator	1974	Hill
Silica-free silicone rubber membranes	1974	Kolobow
Perfusion with minimal anticoagulation	1975	Zapol
Ethylcellulose perfluorobutyrate and polyalkylsulfone	1975	Ketteringham
Permanently implanted booster lung	?	

A major challenge is the design of nonthrombogenic membrane oxygenators that would not require the use of any anticoagulant. This requires consideration not solely of the membrane oxygenator itself, but of the entire extracoporeal circuit. There is increasing evidence that circuits coated with a single surface material, whatever that material may be, fare much better with minimal doses of heparin than circuits assembled of different materials, however well selected. The clinical value of preserving the normal clotting mechanism during the course of long-term perfusions is readily apparent.

The ultimate challenge is to develop a membrane lung that could be permanently implanted in the body. Such a prosthesis could function as a "booster lung" to supplement inadequate respiratory function over prolonged periods of failure, or it could fully replace the natural organ. However formidable this problem might appear, however remote a clinically acceptable solution, the technical challenge of an implantable lung is probably no greater than that of an implantable heart, and the medical need is just as great. History of artificial organs suggests that it takes 10 to 20 years to pass from a working laboratory prototype, even proven clinically, to a device acceptable for clinical use. Remember, for instance, the time lag between the pioneer efforts of W.J. Kolff in hemodialysis in 1943–44 and the advent of maintenance hemodialysis around 1960. Observe the delay between Molopoulos' design of the intra-aortic balloon, and its widespread acceptance in the past few years. An even longer interval separates the pilot clinical application of membrane oxygenation by Clowes and his team in Cleveland, as well as Thomas in Paris, and the generalized use of membrane lungs of the past few years. If the same period of incubation proves necessary with the implantable lung, a clinically acceptable device should be available before the turn of the century.

CHAPTER 6

Extracorporeal Membrane Oxygenation for Acute Respiratory Insufficiency: Current Status

E. Converse Peirce II

Supported by Contract No. NO1-HR-42923 from the National Heart and Lung Institute.

INTRODUCTION

Deaths from or associated with acute respiratory insufficiency (ARI) are variously estimated at 40,000 to 100,000 per year in this country despite important advances in management, especially the more widespread use of well monitored and controlled positive endexpiratory pressure (PEEP).[16,33] Although these figures may be unrealistically high, many cases of ARI occur in all age groups and there is an important peak among newborn infants.[3] Some measure of the patient risk can be gained by looking at statistics of patients placed on ventilators in well-run intensive care units. Data were collected during the latter half of 1975 and early 1976 by nine teams having National Heart and Lung Institute (NHLI) contract support for membrane oxygenation (ECMO). Because our use of oxygen appeared to differ somewhat from other teams, we also studied patients at the Mount Sinai and Bronx Veterans Administration Hospitals receiving less than 50 percent oxygen. The lowest mortality (29 percent) was at the Bronx VA Hospital where perhaps half of the patients were post open heart surgery and given mechanical respiratory support as a matter of policy (Table 1). Cardiothoracic patients at Mount Sinai Hospital are treated in a separate intensive care unit (ICU). Those treated in the general surgical ICU had a mortality of 59 percent. National study patients receiving an FiO_2 of 0.5 for 24 hours or more had a mortality of 76 percent, while the Mount Sinai-Bronx VA patients meeting the same inclusion criteria, had a mortality of 87 percent. Data on perfused patients are given for completeness. The mortality rate was 87 percent in the worldwide group and 92 percent in the NHLI contract group.

The high current death rate of respiratory failure is the result not only of the intrinsically high mortality of ARI patients, despite the expert use of modern intensive respiratory care,[5] but is also a reflection of the severe multiorgan nature of the problems presented. Most primary respiratory failure patients seen at Mount Sinai Hospital had contraindications to ECMO and at least half of the total had other problems more serious than their ARI (Table 2). Only four patients were considered suitable for perfusion. Three of these were perfused and one was a NHLI control. There were no survivors (Table 3).

TABLE 1. Respiratory-Insufficiency-Associated Mortality

	TOTAL NUMBER OF PATIENTS	MORTALITY(%)
12-hr mechanical support		
Bronx VA Hospital, separate ICU	24	29
Mt. Sinai Hospital, separate ICU	88	59
24-hr support FIO_2 0.5		
Total NHLI study*	143	76
Bronx VA Hospital and Mt. Sinai Hospital	24	87
Perfused ECMO		
Worldwide†	233	87
NHLI study‡	36	92

**June–Dec. 1975.*
†Ten years through 1975.[12]
‡May 1974–April 1976. Nonperfused control patients had a similar mortality.

TABLE 2. Distribution of 59 Deaths*

PRIMARY CAUSE	NUMBER OF PATIENTS	%
Respiratory	29	50
Cardiovascular	18	30
Hemorrhage	5	9
Neurological	5	9
Nutritional	2	3

Mt. Sinai Hospital, 8 Months, 1975

TABLE 3. SICU Respiratory Cases*

METHOD	NUMBER OF PATIENTS	SURVIVED
Respirator 24 hrs	112	53 (47%)
Same at Fio_2 0.5	12	1
Perfusion (ECMO)	3	0

Mt. Sinai Hospital and Bronx Veterans Administration Hospital, May–Dec. 1975.

RATIONALE OF ECMO

ECMO is of interest in the management of ARI because the membrane oxygenator, or lung, permits prolonged respiratory support, up to at least three weeks, of patients with minimal lung function.[2,3,9,11,12,16,17,21,23,25,28,40] Other types of oxygenators are so damaging to blood that they may be used safely for perhaps two to four hours only.[26,27] At the blood gas or blood membrane interface, there are important physical forces leading to alteration or destruction of the formed elements of blood and to denaturation of proteins and other large molecules. In a conventional bubble oxy-

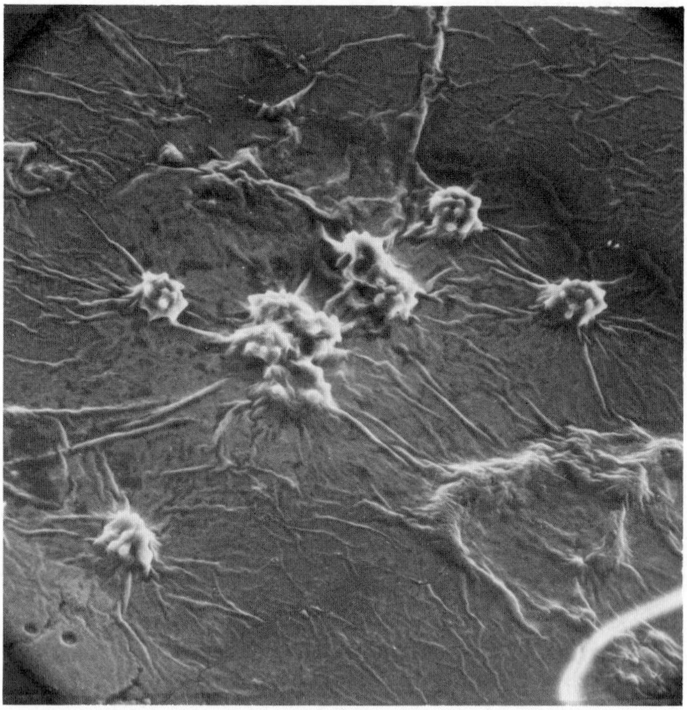

FIG. 1. Scanning electron micrograph of membrane from a General Electric Dualung used for 9 days in a clinical perfusion. The surface is covered by a continuous layer of protein, with some folding probably due to fixation. A number of cells, probably platelets, are seen also (× 1000). (Courtesy Dr. Charles Akers, Calspan, Corp., Buffalo, N.Y.)

genator, damage is cumulative, as everything damaged at the blood-gas interface is plowed back into the flowing blood. In the membrane lung, on the other hand, a protective adherent layer forms at the interface so that blood soon sees a surface largely composed of native protein, and, in consequence, damage is limited (Fig. 1). This is no longer an esoteric theoretical matter, but a proven practicality demonstrated in actual prolonged human perfusions.[27]

The rationale then is to use ECMO to prolong life with the expectation that (a) hypoxia can be reduced, (b) complications, such as pneumothoraces,[36] are made more manageable, (c) iatrogenic damage is reduced by moderation of ventilator pressures, oxygen concentration, and pulmonary artery pressure, (d) concomitant circulatory failure is controlled,[27,37,38] and (e) the reversal of the underlying lung pathology is facilitated.

TECHNIQUE OF ECMO

The technique most successful in accomplishing these objectives is to use a high-capacity membrane lung (of which five or six good disposable types are available)[11,12] and an automated venoarterial perfusion circuit with blood return to the aortic arch or even to the root of the aorta.[23]

Management of the perfusion, including cannulation, is difficult and includes:

1. Proximal and distal cannulation, which is necessary at many sites to prevent ischemia or venous stasis.[17]
2. High-flow perfusion with a minimum of 50 percent of the patient's actual cardiac output. Since outputs are frequently elevated, much higher flows are needed than previously believed.[33]
3. Control of bleeding, especially by meticulous regulation of continuous low-dose intravenous heparin.[18]
4. Development of fail-safe perfusion controls plus close 24-hour perfusion monitoring.
5. Perceptive monitoring of the pulmonary artery and wedge pressures, cardiac output, oxygen transport, and oxygen utilization, in addition to the usual parameters such as PaO_2.
6. Ability and readiness to employ adjunct therapies, such as hypothermia, hyperalimentation, and hemodialysis.

The following must be done while all essential elements of intensive care are continued.

1. Expert pulmonary care nursing, especially regular turning of 180° or more. This last is the essential foundation of good intensive respiratory care.[32,35] It is particularly difficult in a fully monitored patient on perfusion.
2. Continuation of expert mechanical ventilation with optimal PEEP and so forth. Management of the airway may offer formidable problems because high ventilation pressures may still be needed despite perfusion support.
3. Maintenance of nutrition, by hyperalimentation if necessary, is difficult but very important since most patients are hypermetabolic.
4. Application of meticulous measures to prevent and control sepsis. Timely identification of specific pathogens is essential to determine appropriate antibiotics.
5. Fluid management appropriate to the circulatory, pulmonary, and renal status. This is not easy since the requirements for the different organ systems may be quite different.

CURRENT STATUS OF ECMO

Table 4 summarizes worldwide data collected by Gille[11] and by Gille and Bagniewski,[12] plus the results of the first two years of the nine-group National Heart and Lung Institute (NHLI) cooperative study.[28] Diminution in case acquisition and a much lower survival rate than expected have prompted an agonizing reappraisal of the situation. In 1974, the worldwide results looked promising. Twenty-four percent of 167 patients improved sufficiently so that perfusion could be discontinued, and half of these patients survived. The survival rate has not improved significantly worldwide. In the more rigorously controlled NHLI study,

TABLE 4. ECMO Patients

CASES	TO 1974[11]	1974–75[12]	NHLI STUDY*
Number of patients	167	65	36
Improved	40 (24%)	?	6 (16%)
Survived	19 (12%)	10 (15%)	3 (8%)
Number of teams	63	28	9
Number of devices	8	8	5

**Figures for non-perfused random controls essentially the same.*

control and perfusion cases have essentially identical low values for improvement and survival. The full three-year study is not likely to identify a difference.

Infants

A bright spot may be the treatment of infants with ARI originally pioneered by White et al.[40] Optimism is suggested by a recent report of Bartlett et al, showing a 30 percent survival rate for a small group of patients representing a fairly broad spectrum of conditions, several of which are unique to this age group.[3] These data are shown in Table 5. The four patients who survived are clinically well without evidence of respiratory impairment at the present time. Broader efforts are clearly indicated. Unfortunately, the age cutoff for the NHLI study is 12 years, so that the incentive for including infants and children is diminished.

TABLE 5. Respiratory Distress Syndrome in Infants*

DIAGNOSIS	NUMBER OF PATIENTS	SURVIVORS
Post–open heart surgery	2	1
Drowning	1	—
Pneumonia	1	—
Meconium aspiration	4	1
Persistent fetal circulation	1	1
Hyaline membrane	4	1
Total	13	4

**Bartlett et al 1976.*[3]

Correction of Hypoxia

As already indicated, the major objective of ECMO is reduction of hypoxia. On this depends the successful management of complications, such as pneumothorax and the moderation of damage caused by high pressures and high oxygen concentrations. Mechanisms of improving blood gas values during partial cardiopulmonary bypass have recently been discussed by Don et al.[9] The recently compiled worldwide figures of Gille and Bagniew-

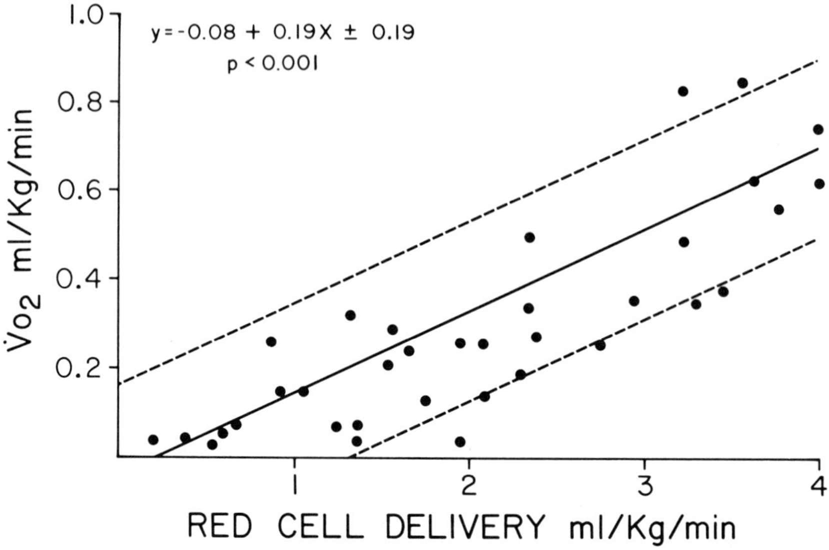

FIG. 2. Dog fish (S. acanthias) perfusion experiment showing a linear relationship between oxygen transport (red cell delivery) and oxygen consumption (VO_2). This is typical of an oxygen conformer. (From Kent et al: Bull Mt Desert Island Biol Lab 15:1975)

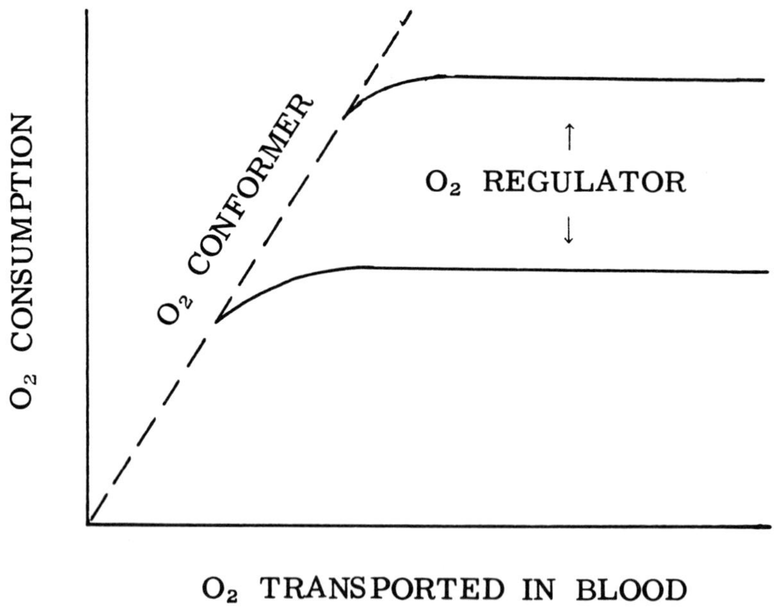

FIG. 3. Diagramatic representation of the relationship between O_2 transport and O_2 consumption for an O_2 conformer and for an O_2 regulator for two different metabolic levels. Healthy man is an O_2 regulator, but hypermetabolic patients with respiratory insufficiency behave as O_2 conformers and increase O_2 consumption without apparent limit as transport is increased.

ski[12] suggest that the PaO_2 was improved in only 59 percent of perfused patients, indicating the possibility of a high technical failure rate. There is even some question of the meaning of the PaO_2 in these perfused patients. We have repeatedly been surprised that a high flow of well oxygenated blood has not permitted us to moderate ventilator settings very much, even though overall oxygen uptake has been considerably increased. Many, perhaps most, ARI patients are hypermetabolic,[15,33] but because of deficient oxygen transport, their high oxygen consumptions are restricted by the low PaO_2, the lower than optimal blood flow, and possibly by tissue transport factors. These oxygen-deprived individuals resemble lower animals who are oxygen comformers (Fig. 2), that is, they adjust their oxygen consumption to environmental and circulatory availability (Fig. 3).[20,34] In these patients, increasing the oxygen transport leads to an increased oxygen consumption to which there is no demonstrable limit (Fig. 4). It is thus not surprising that merely adding a normal basal oxygen exchange via the extracorporeal membrane oxygenator fails to correct the low

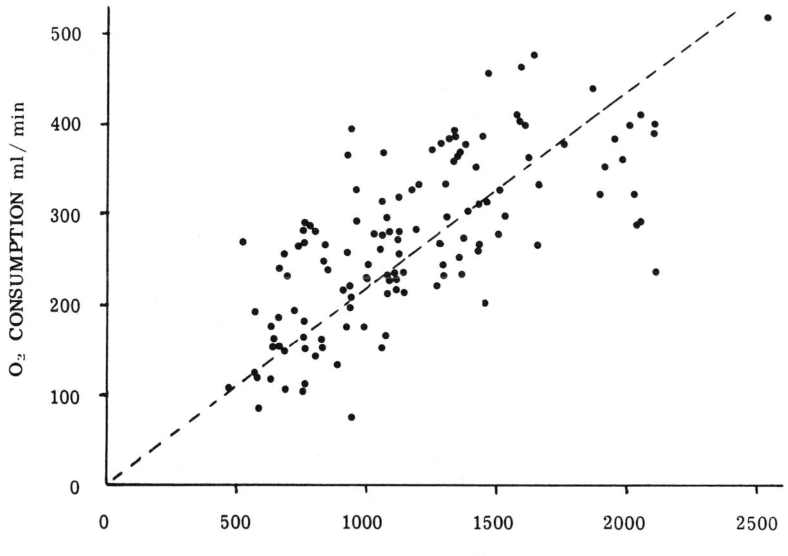

FIG. 4. The relationship between arterial oxygen delivery (transport) and oxygen consumption is illustrated by 126 data points obtained from 33 patients with acute respiratory insufficiency. There is a linear relationship between delivery and consumption with a correlation coefficient approaching one. Clearly, these hypermetabolic patients behave as O_2 conformers rather than O_2 regulators and can use oxygen without any clear limit. (After Powers et al[33])

PaO_2, and so forth. Even if the PaO_2 to the upper part of the body is improved by aortic arch delivery,[23] oxygen needs do not appear to be satisfied. It is likely that hypoxia will need to be assessed on the basis of oxygen delivery and oxygen consumption. As long as the patient behaves as an oxygen conformer, hypoxia probably is still present.

Use of Hypothermia

Very possibly because of difficulties in relieving hypoxia, perfusion hypothermia has been resorted to in one-third of worldwide ECMO cases during the past two years.[12] This modality has been employed with occasional spectacular success in open heart surgery during the past three decades,[24] but has been only briefly considered experimentally for respiratory assistance.[31] Perfusion hypothermia offers remarkable ease in changing or maintaining temperature levels and in controlling the homeostatic temperature regulating mechanism that so often render simple hypothermia difficult to maintain and ineffective in reducing oxygen needs. Several of our cases have appeared to benefit from hypothermia to 31 to 32 C. One case is briefly presented as an illustration. (Data for this case are shown in Fig. 5 and Table 6).

J.M., a 37-year-old male, was admitted in shock on Jan. 16, 1975, for gunshot wounds of the abdomen and left knee. Chest x-ray was read as normal. After volume replacement he underwent multiple small bowel resections, a sigmoid exteriorization, and pelvic drainage. Gastric contents were aspirated from the trachea following intubation for anesthesia. One day later, he bled from his abdominal wound and was given multiple blood transfusions. On the third day, PaO_2 on room air was found to be 35 mm Hg. A chest x-ray showed several rib fractures and diffuse opacification. He was intubated and placed on a volume-cycled respirator, and was at first well maintained on an FIO_2 of 0.5 and a PEEP of up to 15 cm H_2O. He became septic and was treated with antibiotics, diuretics, and colloid. A tracheostomy was performed to facilitate aspiration of secretions. Compliance decreased and PaO_2 gradually fell despite increasing FIO_2. A minute volume of 26 liters was needed to keep $PaCO_2$ within normal limits.

On January 30, 14 days after injury, he met the criteria for slow entry into the NIH ECMO study (PaO_2 50 or below for 12 hours on a PEEP of 15, and an FIO_2 of 0.6 plus a shunt of 30 percent or more) and was randomized to perfusion.

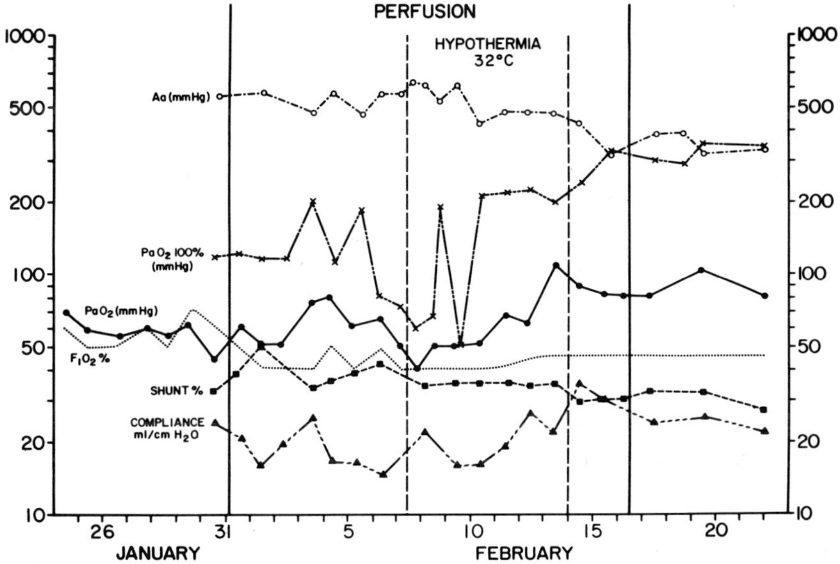

FIG. 5. A 37-year-old male developed acute respiratory insufficiency (ARI) following an abdominal gunshot wound that led to severe blood loss, shock, and probably aspiration. He developed progressive severe respiratory failure and was perfused for nearly 18 days. He failed to improve until hypothermia to 32 C was instituted at the end of the first week. Following respiratory improvement, which persisted, he was weaned from the perfusion but died 6 days later from fulminating Pseudomonas sepsis. Values of special interest are shown in Table 6.

TABLE 6. Values of Special Interest*

	A-a†	Pa_{O_2} 100%†	Pa_{O_2}	Fi_{O_2}	SHUNT†	COMPLIANCE
JAN. 30 Pre–ECMO	551	136	44	.6	.32	24
FEB. 3 Early improvement	432	250	75	.4	.40	24
FEB. 7 Pre-hypothermia	576	74	65	.4	.52	16
FEB. 13 End hypothermia	459	190	115	.45	.35	22
FEB. 15 End ECMO	333	339	80	.45	.30	35
FEB. 19 Best post–ECMO	330	350	110	.45	.32	25

**From top of Figure 5 down.*
†On FiO_2 = 1.0. These values are not exactly concurrent with other values in this table. See Figure 5 for units of measurement.

He was perfused with two 3 M^2 GE lungs by a femoral vein-femoral artery cannulation at about 4 liters/minute. It was possible to reduce PEEP from 15 to 5–10, FI_{O_2} from 0.6 to 0.4–0.45, and minute volume from 26 to 15 liters while Pa_{O_2} rose to 60. Following initial improvement, the condition deteriorated during the first week to about the level of entry. The platelet count fell to less than 50,000. He had recurrent GI, nasal, tracheal, abdominal, and incisional bleeding despite maintenance of activated clotting time at about 150 seconds and generous use of fresh frozen plasma and whole blood. On February 4, he developed a left tension pneumothorax and later a right tension pneumothorax requiring multiple intercostal drains.

Because the patient failed to improve and was hypermetabolic with a cardiac output as high as 8 liters/minute and an oxygen consumption over 400 ml/minute, he was cooled to 32 C. During the second week of perfusion, while cool, he improved dramatically and reached criteria for discontinuing perfusion (Pa_{O_2} of 70 or better on PEEP of 5 and FI_{O_2} of 0.6 or less). The improvement persisted on warming, and he was successfully weaned from perfusion on the 17th day of ECMO. Just before this he was dialyzed once for creatinine of 5.0 associated with high-output renal failure.

He remained stable for 5 days and platelet levels and function returned toward normal. On February 21, Candida was reported from his blood culture, and on February 22, he became hypotensive, anuric, unresponsive to medications, and died. Later a blood culture from February 21 was reported positive for Pseudomonas.

During his illness he received the following:

	WHOLE BLOOD	PACKED CELLS	FRESH FROZEN PLASMA
Before ECMO	19	—	—
During ECMO	31	52	58
After ECMO	—	12	10

Hyperalimentation and antibiotics were used throughout his course, but steroids were given only terminally. An autopsy was performed by the medical examiner. The postmortem findings were as follows:

1. Resolving pneumonia without fibrosis,
2. Severe tracheomalacia
3. Positive lung cultures for Candida, Pseudomonas, and Klebsiella.

No peritonitis or focal intra-abdominal sepsis was found.

Prior to the institution of hypothermia, the patient's condition was deteriorating and respiratory parameters were becoming progressively more abnormal. Although insufficient data are available to show resumption of oxygen regulation, unequivocal improvement occurred concomitant with the hypothermia, and there was sufficient recovery of pulmonary function to permit discontinuation of the perfusion. Perfusion hypothermia appears to offer considerable promise and should be studied both in the laboratory and clinically.

Circulatory Support

The control of circulatory failure by ECMO is very satisfactory,[2,17,29,31] so it is not surprising that conditions such as post–open heart ARI and massive pulmonary embolization are especially responsive to ECMO and have a much better than average prognosis. Pulmonary embolization is a very important form of ARI.[7] Perfusion can reduce mortality without embolectomy. In a small experimental series where perfusion was used on a random basis, four hours of ECMO decreased the mortality from 100 to 60 percent (p less than 0.1).[22,30] A longer perfusion period or postoperative care of the quality available to patients could improve these figures greatly.

Prognosis and Reversibility of Lung Pathology

ECMO patients do, on the average, survive longer than similar patients who are not provided with perfusion support. There are problems (Table 7), especially the risk of hemorrhage and infection, but the prognosis of the perfused patients depends primarily on the reversibility of the underlying lung problem. Where the lung problem is fairly promptly reversible, the results may be spectacularly good. This is true especially of early severe

TABLE 7. Problems Associated with ECMO Patients*

No Improvement	41%
Coagulopathy	34%
Infection	>26%
Hypermetabolism	>33%
Renal failure	>13%

**Modified from Gille and Bagniewski.*[12]

shock lung and of certain opportunistic lung infections where specific therapy is available.[2,12,21] Results are poor in the large group of aspiration and viral pneumonia patients where no specific therapy is known and where early and progressive pulmonary fibrosis frequently occurs.

THE ECMO DILEMMA

Problems of ECMO

Notwithstanding the impression that certain etiologic factors are favorable and others unfavorable, there is no reliable method of selecting patients who are unresponsive to current maximal intensive respiratory care and are likely to benefit from ECMO. In addition, their numbers will be very small for any single institution so that, practically speaking, they must be clearly identified before the timely transfer of such patients to centers equipped to carry out ECMO can occur on a regular basis. Contraindications to ECMO are numerous, especially for the NHLI study, and include brain damage, hemorrhage, terminal cancer, and massive burns. The technique of ECMO is complicated and expensive, especially in terms of personnel. Despite much progress, especially in the control of anticoagulation, the ECMO technique still has only a barely acceptable morbidity and mortality. Perhaps the most important problem, however, is that many potentially reversible lung diseases run too long a course to be effectively influenced by the days or weeks that ECMO can buy. Rather meager studies of surviving ARI patients suggest a continuing slow resolution of pulmonary dysfunction that is measured in months.

WAYS OF IMPROVING ECMO APPLICABILITY

Better Patient Selection

Better patient selection is an imperative. Favorable conditions need to be identified early, before hypoxia has produced irreversible changes. Survivors worldwide have had a mean duration of disease of three days prior to perfusion, while the pre-perfusion duration for failures has been nine days.[12] Improved predictive indices are greatly needed, both for the entire ARI group and for individual diseases.

Bartlett has been most active in developing an overall index based on the value of the A-a gradient (alveolar-arterial diffusion gradient for oxygen) and the duration of the A-a gradient abnormality.[1,4] For this index, the A-a gradient is determined at the ambient FI_{O_2}. Each 100 mm Hg above 300 is coded as 1 and each full day as 1. A patient with an A-a gradient of 500 mm Hg for two days would have a Bartlett pulmonary insufficiency index (PII) of 4. Bartlett has stated that ECMO should be strongly considered in any patient reaching a PII of 3. He has also suggested that the patient is not a good ECMO candidate, and that irreversibility is probable, if the PII reaches 8.[4] In Bartlett's series, collected from five institutions, a PII below 4 carries a chance of survival of 52 percent, while a PII above 4 denotes a chance of survival of only 15 percent (Table 8, p less than 0.001). Although this index considers both severity and duration and represents a very important and useful advance in thinking, there are several major problems. First, the index uses a single physiologic parameter, the A-a gradient, that is influenced by treatment such as the level of PEEP. It may, therefore, not reflect the true severity of the underlying lung disease. Second, the index is greatly influenced by the custom of a particular ICU in choosing the ambient FI_{O_2}. If an FI_{O_2} above 0.4 is used reluctantly, the index may be only a fraction of the value obtained in an ICU where an FI_{O_2} of 0.6 or higher is frequently chosen. Adjusted to the experience of an individual ICU, this PII can be very useful. A more universal index would be obtained at some fixed FI_{O_2} and would probably consider additional variables. The problems of varying the FI_{O_2} in order to collect data, however, can be monumental. For this reason, the shunt fraction

TABLE 8. Bartlett Pulmonary Insufficiency Index (PII)[1]*

INDEX	DEATHS	SURVIVORS
1–4	68 (48%)	75 (52%)
>4	100 (85%)	18 (15%)

**Data represent 261 patients at 5 institutions.* $p<0.001$ *by chi square.*

rather than the A-a gradient may be a better indicator of pulmonary dysfunction. This is notwithstanding the variability of the shunt fraction with the cardiac output, etc, and the problems of obtaining both arterial and mixed venous samples and going to a more complex calculation.

We have observed that failure to increase the PaO_2 with PEEP is a very unfavorable prognostic sign and may well be a contraindication to perfusion since it suggests that destruction of the pulmonary parenchyma by fibrosis has already taken place. We also view progressive loss of compliance, during careful management with an optimal PEEP, as ominous and indicative of progressive irreversibility.

Lung biopsy can be very helpful where the diagnosis of an opportunistic infection is in doubt. In addition, Hill et al have recently attempted to assess the prognosis and the indications for ECMO on the basis of the findings at open lung biopsy.[19] Although they report a positive correlation of fibrosis with mortality in both shock lung and pneumonia, there are as yet too few cases for any firm conclusion (Table 9). Their report is provocative, however, and also documents the very early appearance of fibrosis in many cases both post-traumatic, and infectious as well as the frequent occurrence of fibrin deposition.

TABLE 9. Lung Biopsy*

	NUMBER OF PATIENTS	DIED
Fibrosis	20	17 (85%)
No Fibrosis	16	10 (63%)

**Hill et al, 1976.[19] $p > 0.1$ by chi square*

Unfortunately, we are still too unfamiliar with the natural history of ARI to develop any firm predictors. Some combination of etiology, duration, degree of hypoxia (as measured by the pulmonary shunt fraction and metabolic state, rather than the A-a gradient or PaO_2 alone), circulatory status, and presence of such complications as active air leak, will probably enable ECMO to be selected or rejected on a sound basis. The time for this, however, does not appear to be imminent. ECMO at least has no higher mortality than conventional management as shown by the NHLI randomized study. It is, therefore, clearly ethical to continue studies in this area.

Simplification of Equipment and Procedures

There has seldom been an area in medicine with such visible commercial neglect of small details as long-term perfusion. Only the membrane lungs employed in long-term perfusion circuits represent both a high quality and an appropriate product. Cannulas, devices to secure cannulas, connectors, reservoirs,[8] pumps, bubble traps, access ports, etc, are such a heterogeneous array, it is surprising that long-term perfusion is possible. It is no surprise that perfusions are difficult, time consuming, wasteful of personnel, and frequently a logistic nightmare. Improvements in this area resulting only from application of what is currently known could render long-term perfusion a relatively simple modality that could be easily supervised by a single nontechnical person. The key to improvement is an atraumatic pump that exerts no negative pressure, provides a reservoir function, pumps up to 6 liters of blood at the rate it is delivered to it, and develops a sufficient but safely limited output pressure. These things should be provided on a fail-safe mechanical basis with the potential for prolonged hand operation in an emergency. The experimental Rhône-Poulenc uncaged roller pump fulfills many of these criteria and could be the basis for a modern long-term perfusion system.[10] The so obvious cannula problems need urgently to be met also. A thin-walled, disposable, fully elastic, reinforced cannula, in appropriate lengths and with suitable tips and connectors should not be hard to develop commercially. But who will do it? Finally, the entire circuit should be engineered to eliminate step changes in dimensions and the multiplicity of different materials and joints that makes circuits something of an obstacle course for blood. Solutions to these problems should make much longer perfusions possible.

Specific Therapies for Diseases

ECMO is, of course, not a treatment but a method of prolonging a decision and will be appropriate only to those respiratory conditions that remit spontaneously or that have available specific therapies. The advent of long-term perfusion techniques of low morbidity should encourage collection of data relevant to the natural history of ARI and stimulate development of innovative treatments. It is of interest in this regard that ECMO facilitates the use of pulmonary lavage.[6]

Use of Agents to Prevent Fibrosis

Septic necrosis and fibrosis are the two principal agents of irreversibility in pulmonary disease. The presence or absence of fibrosis can be suspected by pulmonary dynamic changes and documented by lung biopsy.[19] Several agents that may reduce fibrosis by limiting cell division or delaying cross bonding, and consequently maturation, of collagen are available.[13,14] Clinical trials in conjunction with ECMO are already under way at the Massachusetts General Hospital.[41] We have used penicillamine on one occasion very late in the course of radiation fibrosis and plan to use it sooner in future. How rewarding this approach may be is unclear but it deserves consideration.

Lung Transplantation in Terminal ARI

Brief mention of lung transplantation in patients supported by ECMO is appropriate. Vieth has demonstrated the feasibility of transplantation when survival is clearly not possible even with ECMO.[39] Although permanent lung transplantation seems a remote possibility, transplants have been successfully functional for 6 to 10 months. Such a time interval might be sufficient for maximal improvement of the contralateral lung to take place, and patients might then be able to survive after removal of the transplant.

SUMMARY

Extracorporeal membrane oxygenation can prolong life in severe acute respiratory insufficiency (ARI). More than 230 patients have been perfused worldwide for periods up to three weeks with a salvage rate of about 15 percent. Survival has not been shown to be more likely in perfused than in control patients in a small random series developed by nine groups under contract to the National Heart and Lung Institute. The technique of perfusion is difficult, personnel intensive, and has a considerable morbidity. Equipment and techniques urgently need improvement, but the principal unsolved problems are the selection of patients and the lack of specific therapies for most conditions causing ARI. Progress is being made in developing predictive indices that may be used for patient selection, in improving circuitry, and in recognizing innovative concurrent therapies such as lavage and the use of agents to prevent fibrosis. No immediate breakthroughs are predicted, but the field is still a worthy one for those who are determined and not easily fatigued.

REFERENCES

1. Bartlett RH: Personal communication, 1975
2. Bartlett RH, Gazzaniga AB, Fong SW, Burns NE: Prolonged extracorporeal cardiopulmonary support in man. J Thorac Cardiovasc Surg 68:918–31, 1974
3. Bartlett RH, Jeffries MR, Haiduc N, Gazzaniga AB: Extracorporeal membrane oxygenation (ECMO) cardiopulmonary support in infancy. Trans Amer Soc Artif Int Organs 22:80–93, 1976
4. Bartlett RH, Wetmore N, Drinker PA, et al: Indications for extracorporeal membrane oxygenation (ECMO) based on pulmonary insufficiency index. Amer Soc Artif Int Organs Abstracts 5:8, 1976
5. Bryan-Brown CW: Acute respiratory insufficiency: The state of the art. Resp Therapy, March-April:19–25, 1976
6. Cooper JD, Duffin J, Glynn MFX, et al: Combination of membrane oxygenator support and pulmonary lavage for acute respiratory failure. J Thorac Cardiovasc Surg 71:304–8, 1976
7. Dalen J, Alpert JS: Natural history of pulmonary embolism. Prog Cardiovas Dis 17:259–70, 1975
8. Datton RC, Edmunds LH Jr, Hutchinson JC, Roe BB: Platelet aggregate emboli, produced in patients during cardiopulmonary bypass with membrane and bubble oxygenators and blood filters. J Thorac Cardiovasc Surg 67:258–65, 1974
9. Don H, Drinker PA, Hanson EL, Collins JJ: Arterial oxygenation, Mechanisms for improvement during partial cardiopulmonary support. JAMA 228:1419–20, 1974
10. Galletti PM, Richardson PD: Personal communication, 1976
11. Gille JP: L'assistance respiratoire par circulation extra-corporelle avec poumon artificial a membrane. Bull Physiopath Resp 10:373–410, 1974
12. Gille JP, Bagniewski A: Ten years of use of extracorporeal membrane oxygenation (ECMO) in treatment of acute respiratory insufficiency (ARI). Trans Amer Soc Artif Int Organs 22:102–9, 1976
13. Goodman LS, Gilman A: The Pharmacological Basis of Therapeutics, 4th ed, New York, Macmillan, 1975, pp 919–20

14. Gross K, Unholtz K: Therapeutische Beeinflussung der Bindgewebswucherung bei Lungenfibrosen. Pneumonologie 148:201–7, 1973
15. Halmagyi DFJ, Kinney JM: Metabolic rate in acute respiratory failure complicating sepsis. Surgery 77:492–97, 1975
16. Heiden D, Mielke CH Jr, Rodvien R, Hill JD: Platelets, hemostasis, and thromboembolism during treatment of acute respiratory insufficiency with extracorporeal membrane oxygenation: experience with 28 perfusions. J Thorac Cardiovasc Surg 70:644–55, 1975
17. Hill JD: Extracorporeal oxygenation for acute respiratory insufficiency; Clinical experience. Mt Sinai J Med 40:189–98, 1973
18. Hill JD, Dontigny L, de Leval M, Mielke CH Jr: A simple method of heparin management during prolonged extracorporeal circulation. Ann Thorac Surg 17:129–34, 1974
19. Hill JD, Ratliff SL, Parrott JC, et al: Pulmonary pathology in acute respiratory insufficiency: Lung biopsy as a diagnostic tool. J Thorac Cardiovasc Surg 71:64–71, 1976
20. Kent B, Eid JF, Bryan-Brown A, Peirce EC II: Relationships between cardiac output and oxygen consumption in S. acanthias. Bull Mt Desert Island Biol Lab 15:1975 (in press)
21. Kolobow T, Stool EW, Sacks KL, Vurek GG: Acute respiratory failure: Survival following ten days support with a membrane lung. J Thorac Cardiovasc Surg 69:947–53, 1975
22. Krellenstein DJ, Bryan-Brown CW, Geller SA, et al: Extracorporeal membrane oxygenation (ECMO) as a treatment for massive pulmonary thromboembolism. Ann Thorac Surg, in press
23. McEnany MT, Zapol WM, Seebacher J, et al: Cannulation of the proximal aorta during long-term membrane lung perfusion. J Thorac Cardiovasc Surg 70:631–43, 1975
24. Peirce EC, II: Extracorporeal Circulation for Open-Heart Surgery. Springfield, Ill., Charles C. Thomas, 1969, pp 62–82
25. Peirce EC, II: The role of the artificial lung in the treatment of respiratory insufficiency: A perspective. Chest 62:107S–117S, 1972
26. Peirce EC, II: The theory and function of the membrane lung. Mt Sinai J Med 40:119–34, 1973
27. Peirce EC, II: Is the blood-gas interface of clinical importance? Editorial. Ann Thorac Surg 17:526–29, 1974
28. Peirce EC, II: Status of intensive respiratory care for acute respiratory insufficiency. J Maine Med Assoc 67:87–93, 1976
29. Peirce EC, II, Bryan-Brown CW, Lukban SB, Jacobson JH, II, Rothschild JJ: The use of hyperbaric oxygenation in conjunction with membrane lung perfusion for respiratory insufficiency. Mt Sinai J Med 40:228–36, 1973
30. Peirce EC, II, Krellenstein, DJ, Bryan-Brown CW: Blood clots labeled with powdered tantalum for experimental pulmonary emboli. J Maine Med Assoc 67:105–7, 1976
31. Peirce EC, II, Thebaut AL, Kent BB, et al: Techniques of extended perfusion using a membrane lung. Ann Thorac Surg 12:451–70, 1971
32. Pontoppidan H, Geffin B, Lowenstein E: Acute Respiratory Failure in the Adult. Boston, Little Brown, 1973

33. Powers SR, Mannal R, Neclerio M, et al: Physiologic consequences of positive end expiratory pressure. Ann Surg 178:265–72, 1973
34. Prosser CL: Comparative Animal Physiology. Philadelphia, W.B. Saunders, 1973, pp 196–201
35. Ray JF, Yost L, Moallem S, et al: Immobility, hypoxemia, and pulmonary arteriovenous shunting. Arch Surg 109:537–41, 1974
36. Steier M, Ching N, Bonfils-Roberts E, Nealon TF, Jr: Iatrogenic causes of pneumothorax: Increased incidence with advances in medical care. NY State J Med 72:1296–98, 1973
37. Stevens PM: Assessment of acute respiratory failure: Cardiac versus pulmonary causes. Editorial. Chest 67:1–2, 1975
38. Unger KM, Shibel EM, Moser KM: Detection of left ventricular failure in patients with adult respiratory distress syndrome. Chest 67:8–13, 1976
39. Vieth F: Personal communication, 1976
40. White JJ, Andrews HB, Risemberg H, Mazur D, Haller JA, Jr: Prolonged respiratory support in newborn infants with a membrane oxygenator. Surgery 70:288–96, 1971
41. Zapol WM: Personal communication, 1976

CHAPTER 7

Clinical Experience with ECMO: Future Needs

J. Donald Hill

INTRODUCTION

The lung is a fairly reliable organ of the body. In spite of most acute or chronic pathologies, the lung provides a continuous function: It exchanges the body's oxygen and carbon dioxide. With its considerable reserve function, the lung provides necessary respiratory backup. Even in severe pulmonary conditions, improvement of the lung's efficiency and capacity is possible. Raised oxygen content of inspired gas, volume-controlled respiration, PEEP, fluid control, and antibiotics are methods found best to effect this. However, if all these procedures fail, the patient dies.

Therefore, the development of mechanical support for the heart and lungs is an important event in modern medical history. Since it is estimated that almost 75,000 persons per year will die of acute respiratory insufficiency caused by lung disease alone, the technologic mode of extracorporeal membrane oxygenation (ECMO) is a major potential breakthrough in the medical arts.[1]

The history of mechanical support for the heart and lungs is both an old and new story. Old because a bubble oxygenator was employed in the 1880s by Gruber and von Frey. This attempt was followed by a kidney perfusion, by A. Jacobi, using a film oxygenator. However, genuine success had to wait almost a half century before extracorporeal oxygenation became a reality. That event depended on two men: D. McLean for his discovery of heparin in 1916 which made blood incoagulable and J. Gibbon Jr. who created the first mechanical heart-lung machine in 1933. Gibbon's goal was to operate on the heart under direct vision—a revolutionary concept.[2] Although many of Gibbon's colleagues had considered such a procedure, he and his wife made it an actuality, and it worked. The Gibbon machine diverted caval blood to an artificial heart and lung and returned it to the aorta.

The procedure, although relatively common today, continues to be a dramatic one. To date, although many mechanical improvements have been made, the principles inherent in the apparatus are essentially those employed by Gibbon.

Three modes prevailed in the early oxygenators: bubble, screen, and disc. However, they all lacked the ability to effect long-term perfusion. Normally, perfusion time did not exceed six hours. Beyond this time, changes in the blood cell and proteins caused body damage. Although the precise proteins and the nature of the change is not yet clear, it was understood that the basic stumbling block to perfusion was the direct interface of blood and gas. This interface created a surface-free energy that caused a protein breakdown. Early oxygenators were also responsible for hemolysis, which occurred at a rate linear with length of bypass.

The answer to these problems became apparent. A new design was necessary, and the pattern chosen was that offered by the body itself. A membrane that separates the blood and oxygen, simulating the body's mechanism for gas exchange, was incorporated into the oxygenator. The concept of membrane oxygenation resulted. G. Clowes et al were the first to effect the new design by interposing a plastic film between the blood and the gas.

The balance between the blood-flow volume, distribution, and the surface area called for further research and some basic considerations in the design of a membrane oxygenator. Tradeoff and compromise were required: pressure gradient versus transit time, turbulence against blood damage, blood path density versus boundary layer effects. In other words, artificial oxygen and carbon dioxide exchange mandated a more physiological method, one that required sophisticated artificial membranes permeable to the respiratory gases. Longer perfusion times effected today are testimony to the progress in this area.

OBJECTIVES OF ECMO

The objectives of ECMO are simply to accomplish the following.

1. Provide a supplementary gas exchange system for the body to allow the biological lung time to heal using the body's natural mechanism.
2. Provide a more physiological environment which will allow thc lungs thc opportunity to repair themselves.
3. Provide the biological lung with a means of gas exchange support which will allow the application of pulmonary therapy that is otherwise impossible, eg, pulmonary lavage.

SELECTION OF PATIENTS

The problem facing us today is sorting out those patients who have reversible lung pathology. Experience has shown us that many forms of acute respiratory insufficiency are not reversible. Current methods to effect this are not well defined and will be discussed later. Presently, the systemic PaO_2 on a known FIO_2 is the principal method of selecting patients, but its value as an indicator of prognosis and reversibility is very doubtful.

The following are guidelines to the selection of patients.

1. After maximal medical therapy and using optimal respiratory ventilator settings if the PaO_2 is 50 mm Hg while being ventilated with an FIO_2 of 0.6, the patient is a candidate for ECMO.[3]
2. The best results have been obtained in patients who were treated early in the course of the illness. A patient cannot be considered a candidate if the respiratory illness has progressed to 21 days duration. Using current technology, more available data will probably indicate an upper limit of 10 days of illness.
3. Acute and severe hypoxia, myocardial or central nervous system (CNS) depression that cannot be managed using conventional techniques mandate ECMO therapy.

The following contraindications are conclusive.

1. Active bleeding from anywhere in the body is a contraindication for obvious reasons. Patients having controlled hemorrhage (eg, following trauma) can be safely put on ECMO under most circumstances.
2. Irreversible central nervous system damage.
3. Chronic systemic illness, eg, cancer, thrombosis, degenerative central nervous system disease.
4. Evidence of severe left heart failure (left ventricular end diastolic pressure of 25 mm Hg) that is not of hypoxic origin.
5. Acute respiratory insufficiency associated with severe and uncontrolled septic shock and failure of tissue utilization of oxygen.
6. Histological documentation of pulmonary fibrosis.

CANNULATION TECHNIQUES

Three cannulation techniques are generally employed in ECMO, and there are several anatomic sites for their application. Although the most frequently used and advantageous site is the groin (Fig. 1), the neck, the subclavian vessels in the superclavicu-

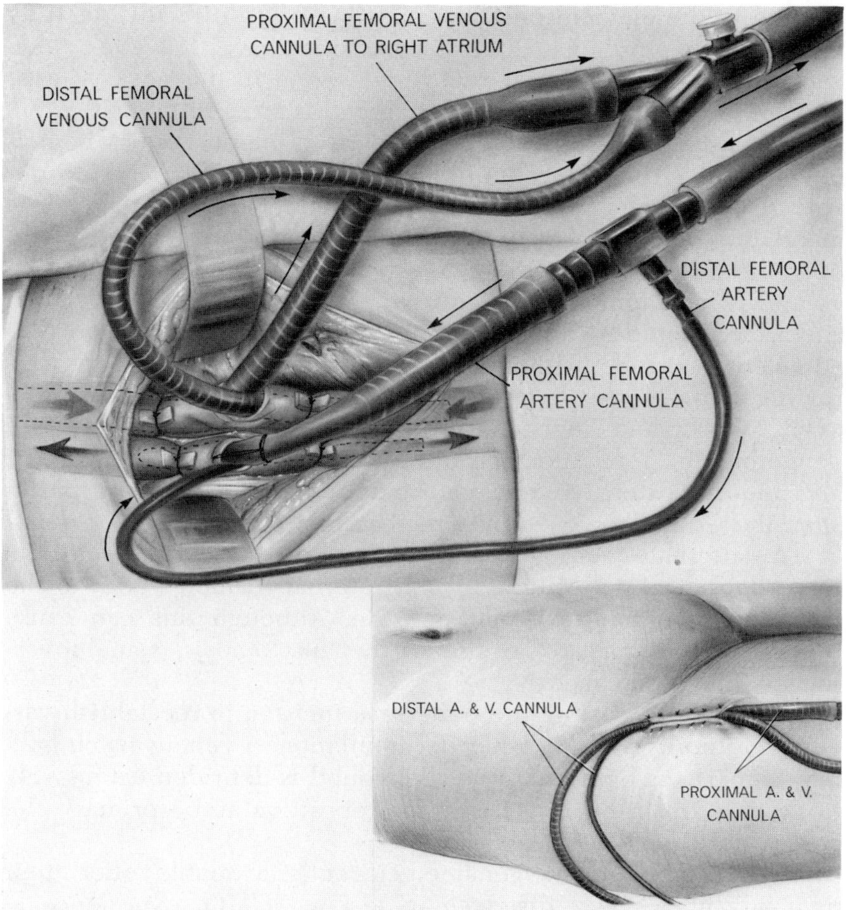

FIG. 1. Details of the arterial-venous cannulation in the right leg.

lar area, and the axillary vessels also serve as cannulation sites. Since on the right, the common femoral, iliac, and inferior vena cava veins are in a straight line favoring introduction of a large thin-walled cannula for venous drainage, the right groin is preferred. It also proves convenient for subsequent nursing care. The one disadvantage of the groin site is its proximity to the genitalia and the potential for wound contamination during perfusion. However, this has not been a major problem.

The axillary vessels are sometimes unsuitable because of inadequate size, and the subclavian vessels have limited accessibility due to the clavicle possibly contributing to difficult bleeding management problems. Both of these sites have, however, been used successfully. The internal jugular vein in the neck is large enough for a satisfactory cannulation and is an excellent site.

Regardless of site, certain surgical principles must be followed at the time of cannulation. Suture transfixion and widespread use of electrocautery provide perfect hemostasis; this is mandatory since anticoagulation with heparin and the inevitable decrease in platelets will cause oozing or bleeding from the wound. Arteriotomy and venotomy are transverse, and the vein and artery should be cannulated proximally and distally to prevent edema or gangrene. Although a vertical incision may risk the narrowing of the vessel lumen, it is an acceptable procedure. However, two separate incisions in either the artery or the vein are dangerous: Ischemic necrosis of the intervening vessel may occur and require extensive revision at decannulation. During perfusion, the wound is closed over the cannula without packs.

An alternate method to proximal and distal cannulation of the artery is that of suturing a 10 mm internal diameter graft to the common femoral artery, end to side. Although this can cause bleeding problems at the site of the anastomosis, some investigators find it satisfactory.

A simple closure of the transverse incision to reestablish vascular continuity accomplishes decannulation. A venous patch graft may sometimes be necessary. The wound is debrided extensively to provide fresh, healthy tissue for apposition and a primary closure is performed.

The membrane oxygenators currently available offer their own advantages and disadvantages. For ECMO, experience at Pacific Medical Center (PMC) has been with the Bramson oxygenator only. It is a fixed volume unit containing an integral heat exchanger, with all perfusions conducted at 37 C. A servomechanism monitors the venous returns, and the pump speed is controlled accordingly.

Two systems of bypass were the standard modus operandi for prolonged perfusion until recently when a third had been added. The first two, venovenous (v-v) and venoarterial (v-a) were combined into the venovenous/venoarterial method, answering the demand for better physiologic values. The venovenous method (Fig. 2) drained the venous blood from the inferior vena cava just below the diaphragm and forwarded it to the membrane oxygenator. The oxygenated blood was delivered to the superior

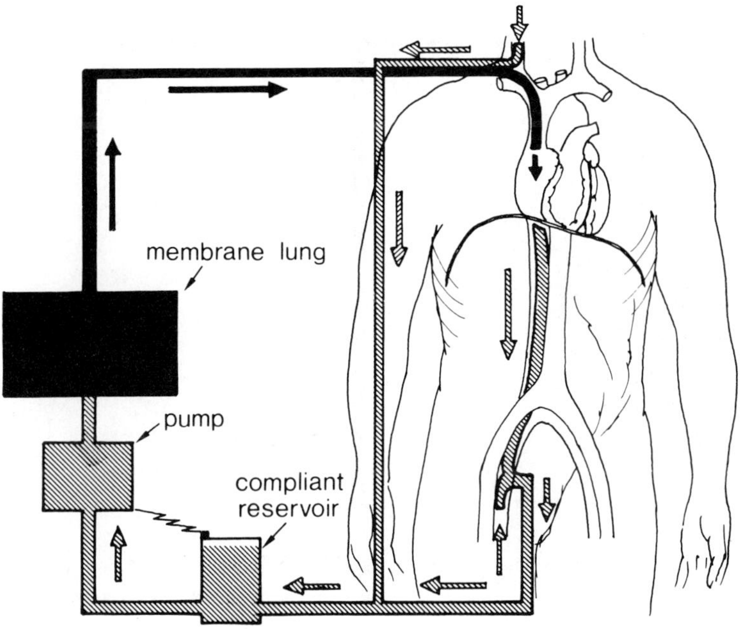

FIG. 2. Cannulation technique: Venovenous bypass.

vena cava via the internal jugular vein. Mixing occurred in the venous return to the right heart, and the entire systemic circulation was supplemented with well-oxygenated blood. With the flow rates, which are necessarily high, the pressures in the pulmonary circuit remained relatively high as well.

Technically, the potential for pulmonary recovery was enhanced by the venoarterial system (Fig. 3), because it reduced pressures in the pulmonary artery and provided a high bypass flow. Oxygenated blood was returned into the femoral artery. The higher region of the thoracic aorta was the site of the mixing of oxygenator and left ventricle outflow. In this mode, the left ventricular blood oxygen tension may remain low despite reduction of cardiac and pulmonary blood flow and pressures provided by this method. The carotid and coronary arteries sometimes received desaturated blood. The cannula delivering oxygenated blood was therefore moved as far as possible toward the aortic root in order to improve the carotid and coronary artery PaO_2. Thus, the modified v-a method gave better flows, perfused the thoracic root with oxygenated blood, and the pulmonary artery pressure was

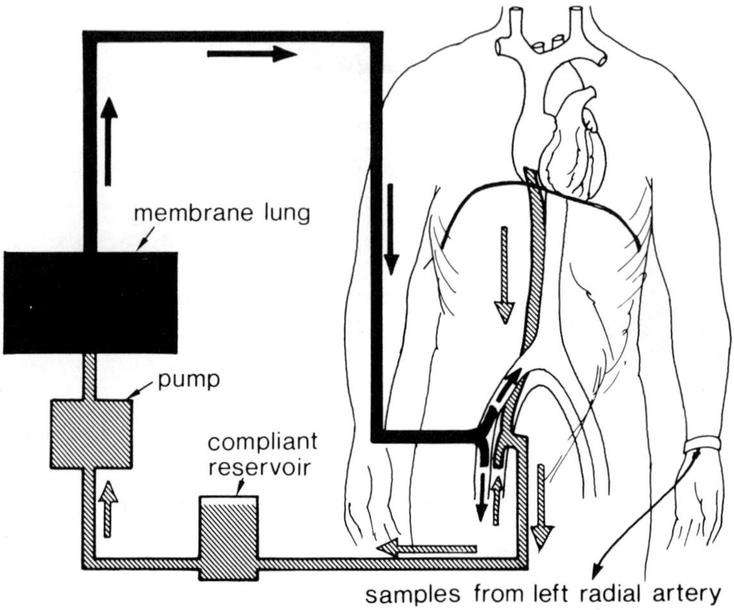

FIG. 3. Cannulation technique: Venoarterial bypass.

substantially reduced. (In some cases, eg, mean pulmonary arterial pressure of 9 to 10 mm Hg, the reduction in the pulmonary artery pressure was so marked, it was believed undesirable for pulmonary parenchymal healing.)

The third system (v-v/v-a, Fig. 4), is technically the addition of a second arterial cannula placed in the right ventricle added to venoarterial perfusion. With the direct return to the right ventricle, a venovenous recirculation loop in the superior and inferior vena cava is not established. This dual technique returns the oxygenated blood to the systemic and pulmonary systems in the ratio of 1:2 to 1:3. A C-clamp controls flow to the right ventricle, which is measured by an in-line electromagnetic flowmeter. The flow is arbitrarily set to give a mean pulmonary arterial pressure of 20 to 30 mm Hg and a saturation of 75 to 80 percent. A compromise is effected between the pulmonary circuit pressure and adequate oxygen supply to the heart and brain. Reduction in ventilatory requirements and systemic pulsatile flow are still maintained.

Determinations of the PaO_2 for all three methods is made from arterial blood samples drawn from an indwelling catheter from

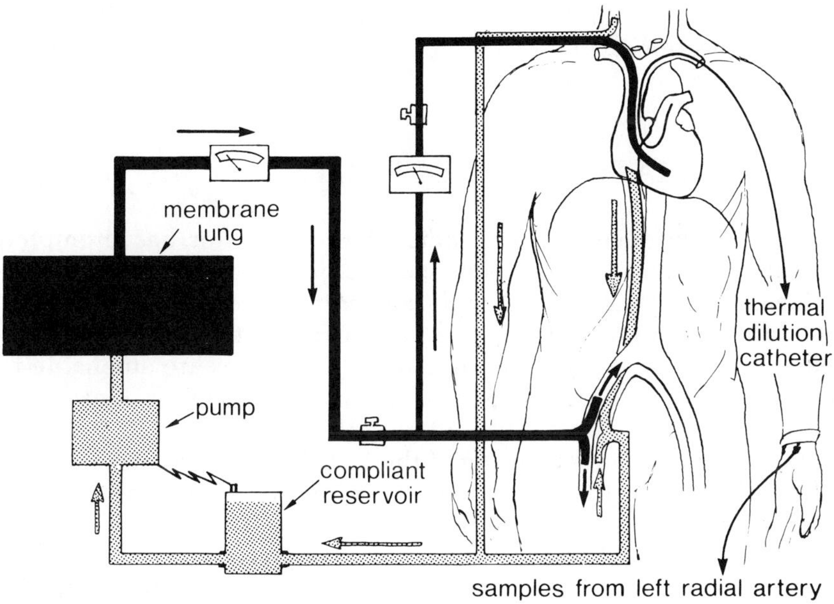

FIG. 4. Cannulation technique: Mixed venoarterial and venovenous system.

either the right or left radial artery. In the venovenous technique, the oxygen saturation in the aortic arch is representative of the entire arterial tree. In the venoarterial system, radial artery blood represents saturation that reached the aortic arch arteries, while employing a high-flow retrograde femoral artery cannulation system. Except perhaps for the coronary arteries, the contralateral radial artery sample will represent the entire systemic saturation if the subclavian artery is used for arterial return. The combined system (v-v/v-a) however, shows the O_2 saturation in the aortic arch with samples obtained from the radial artery. This indicates mixing of already preoxygenated blood from the oxygenator via the pulmonary circuit, with the oxygenator blood delivered via retrograde femoral artery return.

Advancing a #7 French loop catheter from an occlusive sidearm on the femoral artery perfusion cannula determines the exact site of the mixing point in both (v-a and v-v/v-a) modes of bypass as well as LVED pressure and oxygen tension.[4] Blood samples are taken from the left ventricle just above the aortic valve, from the top of the aortic arch, and midabdominal aorta. The gradient in the PaO_2 indicates the height of the mixing point. In any determination of total systemic flow, O_2 consumption, systemic PaO_2, the precise location of the mixing point must be determined if accurate data are to be collected.

HEMATOLOGIC EFFECTS

Experience at the Pacific Medical Center has prompted continuing research into new methods of monitoring the hematological effects of ECMO with concentration on anticoagulation. Bleeding is unquestionably the largest risk in the use of extracorporeal membrane oxygenation. Not all conditions are amenable to the standard methods. The maintenance of long-term extracorporeal circulation mandates anticoagulation of blood in both the patient and machine. Clotting of the blood in the circuitry must be prevented while an effective method of monitoring the heparin level in the patient is maintained.

Lung bovine heparin is used in all bypass procedures. Two methods of monitoring the coagulation time have been used. The Lee-White (WBCT) clotting time and the Hattersley method (activated clotting time; ACT) have been the most acceptable.[5] In the case of the former however, delay in obtaining results and inaccurate reproducibility make it unreliable and unrewarding. In contrast, the Hattersley method has proved to be satisfactory and is used routinely at the Pacific Medical Center.

The Hattersley method can be administered either by hand or by machine at the bedside. In addition, it can be performed by a nurse, physician, or technician and provides rapid, reproducible, and reliable results.[5] Since the ACT procedure is quick, maintenance of a stable state adjusted with heparin is possible even under conditions of changing requirements. Our experience using the Bramson oxygenator has shown that the ACT should be maintained between 180 and 200 seconds. (This is comparable to a Lee-White clotting time of about 30 minutes.) The Hattersley method proved even more constant in patients whose heparin metabolism factors remained steady. This steady state of hypocoagulability required only slight variations in heparin doses.*

Application of ACT to disease states other than those affecting heart and lungs is testimony to its continuing success. These con-

**In order to prevent serious dose-related effects heparin is administered in dilute form (10 percent). A line not employed for anything else is used for infusion into a large vein or extracorporeal circuit using a perfusion pump.*[6]

ditions include disseminated intravascular coagulation, thromboembolism, and renal dialysis.

Recent studies by our group have confirmed a "foreign surface coagulopathy" during prolonged perfusion.[7] This syndrome presents the constant risk of microscopic hemorrhagic or thromboembolic events. To date, causes for the abnormal bleeding are attributed to heparin, thrombocytopenia, and hemostatic incompetence of the available circulating platelets. The regular occurrence of visible oxygenator protein deposition may indicate with more accurate investigation the alteration in the coagulation systems proteins.

Low platelet counts have been attributed to the following: extracorporeal injury followed by destruction in the reticuloendothelial system, splenic or hepatic sequestration, deposition in the injured lungs, and decreased bone marrow production. Yet admittedly, evidence for all these manifestations is both incomplete and conflicting. Platelet survival is shortened (Fig. 5), and in some patients, an active marrow does not preclude continuing decrease in platelet count.[6] Also, any gain in platelets from transfusion is lost very rapidly. Survival times of Cr-tagged platelets were abnormally short. These curves suggest that both young and old platelets are lost, and a more or less uniform mode of injury may cause impaired function.

Since knowledge of the "behavior" of an injured platelet is limited, both platelet injury and qualitative function are difficult to assess. This is exacerbated by the presence of thrombocytopenia and other technical limitations.

Thromboembolic events are ascribed to both systemic emboli, the source of which are the veins of the stiff infected lungs and the embolization of particulate materials formed in the oxygenator. With respect to the latter, platelet microaggregates could be a distinct form. This phenomenon has not yet been confirmed by direct pathological examination, although experiments have revealed that transient microvascular occlusion by platelet aggregates can cause major ischemic damage.

Hemorrhagic disease is also attributable to what appears to be disseminated intravascular coagulation on some occasions. Yet this nomenclature may be worthless to describe a condition occurring in the uniquely artificial situation of prolonged extracorporeal oxygenation. The multiple anticoagulant effects of heparin contribute an uncertain dimension to the actual pathology.

The continual exposure of protein and other formed elements

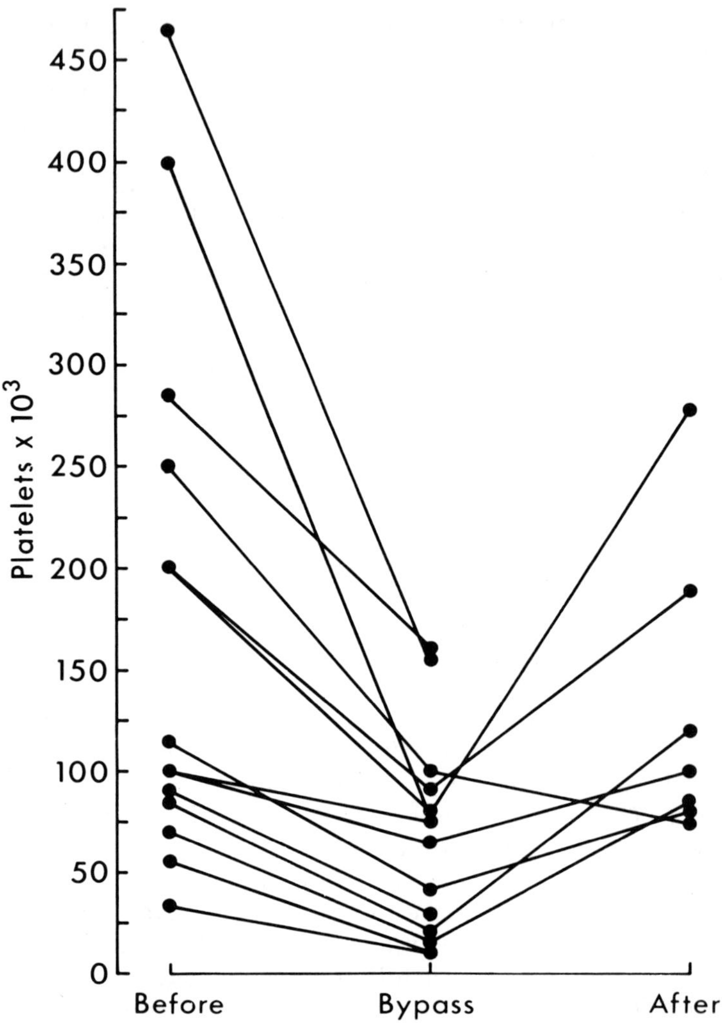

FIG. 5. Platelet levels before, during, and after perfusion.

of the blood to the large artificial polymeric surface and the artificial mechanical stress are perhaps the most difficult problems to interpret. These surfaces adsorb, activate, and denature blood proteins in a way totally without comparison to any activity within the native endothelial environment. Investigators are already aware of the significant curtailment of platelet survival with even minute amounts of foreign surface interposed into the vascular system.

The answer may lie in a different clinical approach using drugs other than heparin for platelet protection and survival. Admittedly, knowledge of the lowest safe level of heparin is still unknown, as is a direct way to measure it. What is suggested is that the minimum level of heparin may be related to that of the circulating platelets and that with few platelets less heparin is required to prevent thrombogenesis caused by the oxygenator.

It must be underscored that platelet transfusions offer little benefit in about a third of our patients in the recent study. They did not control bleeding but they seemed to reduce the general tendency to petechiae that occurs in all body areas when the platelet count reaches 15,000 per mm^3.

Unquestionably, development of better oxygenators will reduce these consequences provided the two critical requirements are met: bland nonthrombogenic materials for areas where blood contacts a foreign surface, and mechanical stresses gentle to the blood. Perhaps the best solution is a 'nonmechanical' one: a pharmacologic blunting of the blood's response.

PROGNOSTIC FACTORS AND RESULTS

Experience and confidence have been gained with the use of ECMO, and the selection of patients for this procedure now has better-defined criteria. The "nothing to lose" aspect of this therapy has been replaced by one supported by experience, data, and literature. Implicit in this is a growing body of knowledge about the selection of patients, the clinical state, and the physiologic features of acute respiratory insufficiency which can mandate the use of ECMO. Even with this, the selection of patients who may have reversible lung disease is the most challenging area for the future.

The following conclusions and data are derived from the treatment of 25 patients at the Pacific Medical Center. The pathophysiologic factors represent a number of disease etiologies.[8,9] In all the cases the principal indication for initiation of ECMO was generalized hypoxemia in the presence of maximum respiratory support, with the clinical observation that the patient was progressing toward irreversible and lethal hypoxemia. Other indications included hypoxemia myocardial or central nervous system depression.

Certain basic criteria for detecting progressive lung failure and determining its prognosis include the following: duration of the illness, pulmonary gas exchange, pulmonary ventilation, renal failure, disseminated intravascular coagulation, and lung biopsy.

Duration of Illness

The duration of time a patient has acute respiratory insufficiency before ECMO is instituted is important in the ultimate prognosis. The range of duration of illness in our study was 5 hours to 24 days. Reviewing the variation in time and final outcome convinced us that patients with a short severe disease course are better candidates than those in a subacute state for whom perfusion is not begun until 12 to 14 days into the course of the disease. The optimum time will probably evolve to be of 1 to 3 days duration.

Pulmonary Gas Exchange

A system was developed to measure pulmonary gas exchange characteristics. This was aimed at determining if the resulting arterial hypoxia was due more to a fixed shunt abnormality (Qs/Qt) or to a ventilation perfusion abnormality (V/Q). Patients with severe hypoxia related to V/Q abnormality had a better prognosis than those having a fixed shunt.[7]

Pulmonary Ventilation

Hypercapnia is never present prior to ECMO therapy. It occurs in patients after ECMO begins however. Progressive lung failure develops and some patients develop major bronchopleural leaks while others progress to destruction of lung parenchymal tissue. Thus a poor overall prognosis is synonymous with the inability to control carbon dioxide. This however is usually not known until one has begun ECMO therapy.

Renal Failure

Renal failure is often associated with ARI. However, renal failure is not an important factor in prognosis since dialysis is easily performed during ECMO, after which the patient requires a vascular shunt. During dialysis, management of cardiopulmonary status is sometimes difficult because of rapid fluid shifts. To avoid major alterations in fluid and electrolyte management, dialysis is performed daily. Anuria reduces heparin requirements.

Disseminated Intravascular Coagulation

Disseminated intravascular coagulation (DIC) is not a contraindication or a poor prognostic sign unless its underlying cause is uncontrollable. Failure reflects inability to control the underlying stimulus to the consumption of the clotting parameters, eg, infection. Eight of our patients presented this syndrome; all but one had DIC before ECMO began. Half of them had satisfactory reversal during perfusion, but in three patients, DIC was partially responsible for the death of the patient as a result of either bleeding or inadequate peripheral circulation.

Lung Biopsy

Open lung biopsy is a new tool which provides an excellent means of diagnosis in ARI.[8,9] Correlation between the gross appearance of the lung at operation and the microscopic findings is good. In addition to its effectiveness, the procedure is safe. In 42 patients biopsied during the acute stage of illness, the mortality was zero, the moribidity only 4 percent. In one-third of the patients, specific diagnoses or therapies were employed as a direct result of the biopsy. Since it is known that knowledge of the early pathophysiology of the disease can give a better insight into possible reversibility of its course and the eventual success of ECMO, the lung biopsy is an excellent tool to be used early in the course of ARI.

The gross appearance of the lung revealed the underlying pathology on many occasions.

Two-thirds of these patients had fibrin or fibrinogen debris in the lung vessels detected by immunofluorescent techniques. Fluorescent hyaline membranes were present in nearly all the alveolar linings. Noteworthy and surprising to our investigators was the abundance of fibrin and fibrinogen immunofluorescent materials in the lung concentrations in the alveoli and aveolar walls. This was not accompanied by a bad prognosis. The most ominous sign was the presence of early or established fibrosis (Fig. 6). The

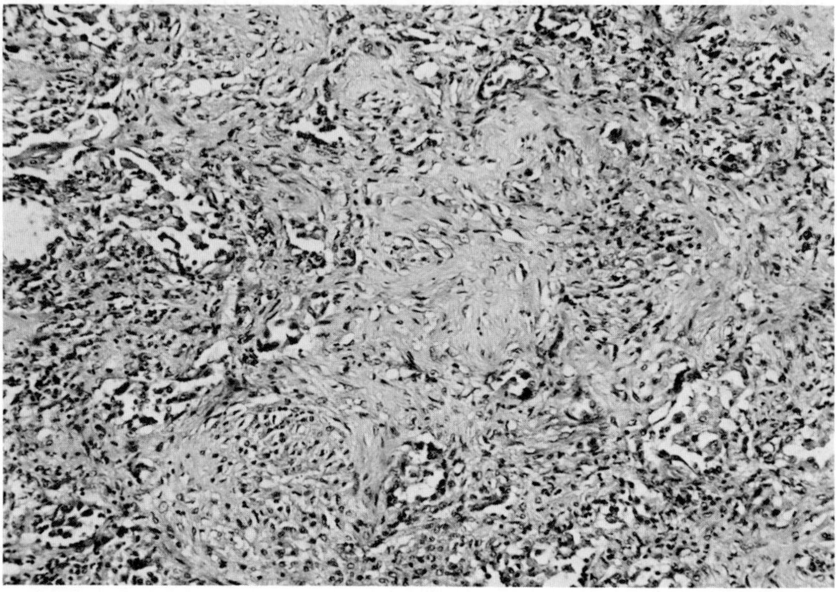

FIG. 6. Diffuse fibrosis as seen in lung biopsy.

mortality rate can be very high (greater than 85 percent), but the chances for survival of trauma patients with fibrosis exceeded that of those with pneumonia and fibrosis. Since the development of fibrosis is synonymous with a poor prognosis, the advantage of open lung biopsy is further underscored. (Fibrosis occurring late in the disease's course is a contraindication to ECMO.)

Detailed description of clinical results of ECMO, lung biopsy, hemodynamic effects of cannulation technique and hematological effects are described in the literature.[9–11]

FUTURE NEEDS

The overall survival rate at PMC and the worldwide results are 15 percent in 1976. How can we improve these in light of current successes?[12]

Although extracorporeal oxygenation is now an acceptable modality for treatment of acute respiratory insufficiency as well as an important adjunct to open heart surgery, its success does not preclude continual experimentation, study, and research into its improvement and expanded use.[13]

Bleeding still continues to be a problem with ECMO. Its current rates show a 15 percent mortality. The answer to this problem lies in new antithrombogenic materials and good in vivo animal tests followed by clinical investigations. Unquestionably, better oxygenators that can prevent the mechanical stresses promoting thrombogenesis are mandatory. But here too, the pharmacologic agents employed play an important part in the success of the therapy. In the case of the latter, the most urgent consideration is the use of heparin. Its contribution to loss of hemostasis must be a major consideration with possible elimination of its use. This can only be accomplished through better assay of in vivo heparin activity by quantitative biochemical tests. Hopefully, a few years will see substrates available to measure clotting factors simply and directly in a wide variety of coagulation components which can provide precise factor concentrations.

Reversibility of lung injury in acute respiratory failure is another major problem of long-term perfusion. Pulmonary fibrosis may destroy the lungs. Therefore more work on lung biochemistry, hematology, microcirculation, and neural influences is necessary to determine lung pathophysiology and better patient selection. Better understanding of the trauma response with respect to age is an important component for improved ARI therapy.

Currently, two solutions to acute lung disease irreversibility have been offered. One is lung transplantation, the other is an implantable mechanical lung. Being mechanically oriented for the future, I choose the latter, but as a physician, I have seriously considered clinical transplantation. However, the problem of rejection must be considered, and this requires a thorough laboratory investigation with the goal of a clinical lung transplantation in selected, irreversible acute lung injury. The biggest obstacle to clinical transplantation at this time in these patients is the universal presence of bacterial organisms in the recipient tracheal bronchial tree.

The outlook for ECMO continues to be good, and we now know that there are certain classes of ARI patients in whom a high salvage rate is possible. These include early trauma with severe hypoxia, severe ARI post–open heart surgery, pulmonary blood and fat emboli, and opportunistic infections. But these problems must be investigated one at a time. In addition, it must be remembered that the most efficacious treatment is early prevention. More information in this area will parallel improvements in ECMO technology.

REFERENCES

1. Hill JD: Prolonged extracorporeal circulation. In Ionescu MI (ed): Current Techniques in Extracorporeal Circulation. London, Butterworth, 1976, p 517
2. Bartlett RH, Harken DE: Instrumentation for cardiopulmonary bypass—past, present, and future. Medical Instrumentation 10:2, March, April 1976, p 119
3. National Heart and Lung Institute, Protocol for *Extracorporeal Support for Respiratory Insufficiency,* Collaborative Program. May 15, 1974, p 3
4. Hill JD, Gerbode F: Prolonged extracorporeal oxygenation. In Sabiston D Jr, Spencer F (eds): Gibbon's Surgery of the Chest. Philadelphia, Saunders, 1975, p 872
5. Hattersley PG: Activated coagulation time of whole blood. JAMA 196:436, 1966
6. Heiden D, Mielke CH, Rodvien R, Hill JD: Platelets, hemostasis, and thromboembolism during treatment of acute respiratory insufficiency with extracorporeal membrane oxygenation: Experience with 28 clinical perfusions. J Thorac Cardiovasc Surg 70:651, 1975
7. Lamy M, Fallat RJ, Koeniger EL, et al: Pathology and mechanisms of hypoxemia in adult respiratory distress syndrome. In: Zapol W, Orist J (eds): Artificial Lungs for Acute Respiratory Failure, New York, Academic, 1976
8. Fallat RJ, Lamy M, Koeniger EL, Hill JD: Use of physiologic and pathologic correlations in evaluating ARDS. In: Zapol W, Orist J (eds): Artificial Lungs for Acute Respiratory Failure, New York, Academic, 1976
9. Hill JD, Ratliff JL, Parrott JC, et al: Pulmonary pathology in acute respiratory insufficiency (ARI): Lung biopsy as a diagnostic tool. J Thorac Cardiovasc Surg 71:1, 65, 1976
10. Hill JD, Ratliff JL, Fallat RJ, et al: Prognostic factors in the treatment of acute respiratory insufficiency with long-term extracorporeal oxygenation. J Thorac Cardiovasc Surg 68:6, 1974
11. Eberhart RC, Lamy M, Dietrich HP, et al: Hemodynamic aspects of prolonged extracorporeal oxygenation. Trans Am Soc Artif Int Organs 1974
12. Gille JP, Bagniewski AM: Ten years of use of extracorporeal membrane oxygenation (ECMO) in treatment of acute respiratory insufficiency (ARI). Presented at 1976 meeting, Am Soc Art Int Organs, San Francisco. Transactions ASAIO 22:102, 1976
13. Hill JD: Horizons: Present problems in applications of ECMO to acute respiratory insufficiency. In: Zapol W, Orist J (eds): Artificial Lungs for Acute Respiratory Failure, New York, Academic, 1976

Discussion

MEMBERS OF PANEL

HENRIK H. BENDIXEN, M.D.
Moderator

PIERRE M. GALLETTI, M.D.

J. DONALD HILL, M.D.

E. CONVERSE PEIRCE, II, M.D.

WARREN M. ZAPOL, M.D.

Dr. Bendixen: Let me first say that we will start with a question that can be directed to all three speakers.

If you had to name one patient who would be the foremost candidate for extracorporeal membrane oxygenation, who would it be? Dr. Hill?

Dr. Hill: The foremost candidate for ECMO? Well, as a group, I would say trauma patients with shock lungs, and specifically, who have a problem with capillary leak syndrome, in which the lung architecture really has been preserved, but the patient is severely hypoxic and you cannot manage him by conventional means. He is probably the best.

Dr. Peirce: Post-trauma patients, where pulmonary edema is the major factor. I think I am saying what Dr. Hill said, because what you want is something that is clearly reversible.

You want a pathology for which buying a little time will provide a chance for the lung to recover, and this is the type of thing that we have the greatest success with.

I would put the pulmonary emboli in there somewhere. The problem with these patients is to get to them early and decide which ones are going to die if you don't do something. I think you could salvage most pulmonary emboli patients with this technique.

Dr. Bendixen: Do you agree?

Dr. Zapol: I would agree, yes. I would stretch it out and say that I think that a reasonable number of post-trauma patients are really patients with infection, and that's why they get into their pulmonary problems.

I think we are into the stage beyond microembolus infusion. These probably don't trouble me so much.

As long as you have a pretty good idea that is what you are dealing with, then you can work with it.

Dr. Bendixen: What would be the worst patient you could think of, Dr. Hill?

Dr. Hill: The person that has had viral pneumonia 15 days, and comes with an FIO_2 of one and chest tubes on both sides with air leaks and secondary infection on top of it. These are the kind of patients that I get referred, and in five years, regardless of what treatment I have used, there has been one survivor.

Dr. Bendixen: You are paraphrasing someone else's failure; is that it?

Dr. Peirce: I would only add to that. I think it is a very bad prognosis if you get no improvement when you use positive end expiratory pressure. These are the patients with fixed shunts. Patients who don't respond to positive and expiratory pressure are pretty much hopeless.

Dr. Zapol: I go along with viral pneumonia. I would separate out varicella however since both Dr. Edmonds and myself have had good results in treating the latter. I would separate out two patients I had that resulted with that.

I would suggest that influenza (A type A and A_2) is probably the worst offender, and we have grown that large number of cases, all of whom have done terribly.

Dr. Bendixen: Let's go next to some specific questions. Here is one that I would like some references and some discussion of: What can you do to combat pulmonary fibrosis? First of all, to what extent is this a problem and can you give an explanation for it?

Dr. Zapol: I think we have to go to what the pathologist tells us when he slices the lung. He sees a large number of alveoli that are obliterated with fibrous tissue and alot of interstitial fibrosis and I think you have to agree that probably that is a severe problem.

There has been very little work with quantitative morphology in either animals or in man, but what little there is tells us that there is an increase in the collagen in the lung. It is only about a 10 to 20 percent total increase in collagen, but it is definitely there.

Recently, in the last six months or so, we have looked at the microscopic distribution of collagen, and what happens is that the lung redistributes itself. It redistributes its collagen away uniformly splattered about the lung to right into the middle of the alveoli, and breaks it down all over.

Sick lungs break down and build up in the wrong places. What can you do to block it? There are at least three very potent collagen blocking drugs, none of which can be used in humans.

There is a tiny amount of knowledge about the use of β-amino proprionitrol in rats by Levine, which shows that the drug blocked pulmonary collagen accumulation in rats. That is the only data there is, and I believe it is a relatively benign drug.

We have used β-amino proprionitrol which is a lysol oxidase inhibitor. It inhibits the cross-linking of collagen. The collagen that's secreted is soluable and can be carried away. We've used it five times, two times late in viral pneumonia, once somewhat earlier in a viral pneumonia staph-infected and more recently in two patients who had open lung biopsies. One patient had diffuse interstitial fibrosis and nodular pattern. He recovered and went home after three weeks of BAPN. The other patient is a young girl who is still in the hospital and is considerably improved.

Dr. Bendixen: Thank you. There are several questions here having to do with dehydration nutrition.

Dr. Peirce, would you like to start out and tell us what you aim at when it comes to supplying calories?

Dr. Peirce: Well, we think that most of these patients need to be hyperalimented and one of the earliest things that we do is to put them on a hyperalimentation regimen similar to any other patient who is starving, because these patients are basically starving.

I think this has not been a routine procedure across the board with other groups.

In terms of fluids, obviously, one has somewhat divergent demands of the different organ systems in the body.

We are interested in what goes on in the lung. We are interested in what goes on in the vascular compartments. We are interested in what goes on in the kidney.

They may require quite different fluids at any particular moment. If we give too much fluid, we are likely to aggravate pulmonary edema, if we give too little, we are likely to end up with too small a blood volume.

We do use colloids. We are rather vigorous with the treatment of colloids. We believe it is the safest fluid to augment the blood volume, and that water should be given primarily to replace renal fluid loss and insensible loss. It requires a good bit of judging. I think ideally, these patients should be weighed daily. We have not been able to effect this clinically in our particular setup.

I think that this should be done, and I think that one needs to set up a very careful balance sheet and to be very careful not to feed too much free fluid.

Dr. Bendixen: This obviously is important, so let me ask Dr. Hill, do you have any different approaches to this problem?

Dr. Hill: Not really. It has been suggested in the beginning, in around 1970, before we had an appreciation of the importance of nutrition, we did not hyperaliment these patients. But now we use it in all patients.

Dr. Zapol: I have nothing on that.

Dr. Bendixen: Dr. Peirce, there is some interest in your concern with the metabolism and the cooling. Would you say a little bit about that? Do you cool all your patients?

Dr. Peirce: You can reduce the metabolic requirement of the patient considerably.

Of course, if you reduce the temperature, and at the same time eliminate the thermoregulatory control. If you don't regulate the thermocontrol, you can actually increase the oxygen demand, so it has to be done very carefully.

Eliminating even imperceptible shivering depends upon the patient. This is simple or difficult.

With the patients that we have on perfusion it is extremely easy, because we provide the cooling with the perfusion and it is very easy to overcome their thermoregulatory mechanisms.

Also, most of these patients are more or less paralyzed. They are, at least, heavily sedated, so that it has not been difficult to reduce their oxygen requirements.

Our data are not good and I don't have the kind of figures to show to you that, for example, we can predict that if we take a patient to 32 C, this will reduce his oxygen need by 35 to 40 percent and this is exactly what happens.

Our data are much more scattered because of the problems of collecting oxygen consumption data in these very sick patients, but the trend appears to be considerably reduced oxygen consumption, and in some of the patients, it seems to follow the pattern of prediction very well.

The patient that I mentioned in whom we had really rather dramatic improvement in the clinical condition where the cooling had not been apparent in an entire week of perfusion prior to that time, is very strongly suggestive, but again, it is not the kind of thing that is conclusive. This is a neglected area.

Hypothermia was very popular in the fifties and for a couple of years in the sixties, and now it has largely been abandoned. I think it has been abandoned by people who call it hypothermia.

Cardiac surgeons use it every day, but it is not called that. It is coming back now, and I think we will be a little more astute about using it and will find that it is a measure that will greatly reduce the oxygen needs in patients, and therefore, will be very helpful.

I personally think that it is probably one of the basic treatment techniques that should be used, and we have used it in some of the patients even without perfusion and it seems to be helpful.

Dr. Bendixen: One of the traps in surface cooling, of course, is shivering, and there is nothing in this world that can increase metabolism more than shivering.

What would you specify as a way to avoid shivering in these patients?

Dr. Peirce: Well, all of these patients are on mechanical respiratory support and most of them require some heavy sedation. We have usually used morphine and Pavulon, and when we have even the vaguest suggestion of shivering or hypermetabolism, we add chlorpromazine, and this appears to be effective.

Dr. Bendixen: What about Dr. Zapol, are you cooling, and Dr. Hill, are you cooling, and if you are, are you using the same technique, and if you are not, why not?

Dr. Hill: We never cool except under one circumstance, which ultimately tells you something else. That means after seven, eight or nine days of bypass, you slowly start to have a problem with CO_2, which probably means that your lung, the biologic lung, is being destroyed, and we may cool a little bit, but never really much below 34 C and most of the time we perfuse at 37 C.

Dr. Zapol: We routinely, I would guess, perfuse between 32 C and 34 C. We do not use a heat exchanger.

Dr. Bendixen: I am not sure I caught you.

Are you saying that you end up cooling because of all of the things you do, or do you do it deliberately?

Dr. Zapol: We routinely cool, and we routinely want to keep people reasonably cool.

Dr. Bendixen: All right. And several questions have to do with the circulatory state. Are you taking steps to support the heart with such things as digitalization? Are you measuring cardiac output and what is your endpoint with respect to cardiac output? Dr. Hill?

Dr. Hill: Well, we don't give digitalis. We used to at one time, but we just stopped doing it. It did not make a difference.

Most of these patients have good strong hearts before they have ARI, so we haven't noticed that left ventricular failure is a particular problem.

We measure cardiac output with thermodilution techniques. We don't have any great guidelines, whether or not we would like to see it at a certain level.

We measure wedge pressures but don't pay a lot of attention to them, not because we don't believe in that measurement, but it is just that in ARI patients, we found them to be grossly abnormal most of the time because of the pathology in the lung. If we think we have a left ventricular problem, we pass a catheter retrograde and measure the LVEDP and make our adjustments accordingly. Other than that, on bypass most of the time we would be bypassing somewhere around 3 liters, I would say.

Dr. Bendixen: What is your endpoint?

Dr. Hill: My endpoint would be that I want to have a sufficient bypass so that I can reduce the FiO_2 setting to around 0.5 or 0.4, maintaining PO_2 in the 60s, and then I am satisfied, especially if we could also reduce the mean trachial pressures and total volumes.

Dr. Peirce: Well, most of us, of course, use venoarterial support, and this provides a considerable boost to the circulation and helps the failing heart. Many of the patients with acute respiratory insufficiency have failing hearts prior to the perfusion and this support may be beneficial—there may be a dramatic improvement with the perfusion. We have seen this particularly in patients who have post-openheart respiratory insufficiency, coupled with a low output syndrome.

The perfusion is very supportive. We don't have any particular endpoint, but we worry about patients who, on perfusion, (say 3 to 5 liters a minute), still have cardiac outputs in the order of 5 liters a minute or more.

This is of considerable concern, and we would like to see the cardiac output lowered, but we don't always seem to be able to get it down.

Dr. Bendixen: Do you use digitalis?

Dr. Peirce: Not routinely.

Dr. Bendixen: Dr. Zapol.

Dr. Zapol: Let's simply say that I think a FIO_2 below 50 percent, peak ventilator pressure below 50 cm H_2O, and a PO_2 in the 50s and 60s are fine. I would consider those practical endpoints.

I would just like to think about the heart for a moment. I would like to maintain pulmonary blood flow to a point where the PVR is acceptable. You can write out for any patient a PVR index curve and I will maintain him until he plateaus, because at that point he has recruited what he can (the rest is obstructed and won't recruit).

Now, what about the heart in ARI?

We managed right ventricular ejection fractions in the last 15 patients.

We managed their volume status by the right ventricular end

diastolic volume index (index per meter^2), and we run most people between 90 and 100 ml/meter^2 in their right ventricle.

Ejection fractions are down in about 60 percent of patients with ARDS—they tend to be patients with a viral pneumonia—they have a viral myocarditis associated, I suspect.

They usually need inotropic support (Isuprel, etc.). If you look at the right ventricular stroke work index in ARDS, it is three or four or five times elevated in these people.

Clinically, what do I worry about?

I have seen atrial fibrillation three times in the last year. I have seen one 22-year-old girl with a right ventricular infarct. I think that there is a lot of right ventricular work in these people.

We tend to digitalize them, give them inotropes, and worry about their right ventricular function.

Dr. Bendixen: You said in most of these patients, Dr. Hill, that they mostly have young, strong hearts. That brings up something that we haven't mentioned, but I assume that we are all thinking about. The one patient you would not want to select for this would be the old patient?

Do you have any age limits?

Dr. Hill: Well, there are age limits in this study that we are on, which are between the ages of 12 and 65, but frankly, if the person had the right indications and you really thought that with the bypass you would gain on a patient, I would not have any objection to bypassing a patient up to the age of 75.

I would not take somebody who is very risky, but with something to gain, age is not a contraindication per se.

In terms of their heart failure what Dr. Zapol says is true. Viral patients tend to have more of a problem than the others, and other patients have a problem with the ventricle before they are bypassed. But once they get oxygen, the ventricle comes around quite nicely.

Dr. Bendixen: There are several questions about the oxygenator, and people would like to know the problems you have with them. One question has to do with debubbling.

Dr. Zapol: With the spiral coil lung, I would say that the most difficult thing in the long run, is the manifold. But you can see the manifold and you can see how many thrombi are developing.

I guess you have to say the Achilles' heel of our ECMO setup is the manifold. The second problem, debubbling, is, I think, a resolvable problem. If you handle it and CO_2 prime as the manufacturer suggests, you can use a vacuum prime and it works very nicely. Prime in a vacuum and you won't have any bubbles!

Dr. Bendixen: We have several questions dealing with platelets.

Dr. Hill, when you have a patient on EMCO, and things are going well, what kind of platelet count would be acceptable to you?

Dr. Hill: I would accept anything over 40,000, and I don't get really too nervous until they get to 20,000, and even then, I don't really get too nervous unless the patient has some kind of a bleeding problem. I don't like to see a patient blossom out with petechiae, because if it is happening on the skin, it is happening everywhere else.

Dr. Bendixen: What do you do with the very low platelet counts when you do get nervous?

Dr. Hill: I call the blood bank and I say that I want 12 units of platelets, and what I do is to give them platelet packs, and in order to get the platelet count up to 40 or 50,000 and keep it there, you would probably have to give the patient at least 12 to 16 units per day.

You may, however, only have to do that for a day or so, and then the patient will level off in the end.

Dr. Bendixen: If you see petechiae, how do you know that that is not just an accidental correlation with a low platelet count? There are many other possible causes.

Dr. Hill: There are, but the fact is that experience has shown that when you give the platelets, that the petechiae problem tends to disappear.

Dr. Bendixen: Here is another question for Dr. Hill. What membrane are you currently using? Is that defined by the study you are in?

Dr. Hill: It is defined by the study that I am in. I am using the Bramson membrane oxygenator, the one we used from the beginning, and I have been satisfied with it. It has a couple of big potential problems, which we have been working on.

The basic problem is that it has too big a surface area to eventually be a great ECMO support system. What I think is important is to get a system that has a small surface area, then you can put any surface on and be able to go without worrying about bleeding problems. We are now working with a 6-meter^2 system that has a blood screen in it that makes up another 5 meters, so you are talking about a 10-meter^2 surface area.

You cannot help having alterations in blood when dealing with that volume. That is what I am using now, but what I am planning to use and develop is something that has a surface area of 0.6 meter^2, and has a transit time across the oxygenator of 0.3 seconds.

Dr. Bendixen: What causes that disappearance of pulmonary capillaries, and could it have something to do with the tubing, the equipment you are using, and so forth? Is it a disease process or is it secondary to the breakdown of the support system?

Dr. Zapol: If we use veno-arterial perfusion to plug the pulmonary arteries, it would seem that you would have to directly enter the bronchial arteries. I don't think there is enough evidence to show that in man, even in acute lung disease that could wipe out the pulmonary vascular tree.

We see it as well in controlled managed patients that don't have ECMO.

I would suggest that it is the disease process, and we don't know enough yet to see how the vasculature is destroyed. It has to do with the increases in the interstitial pressure in the lungs. The capillaries either plug off or clot. Whatever they do they disappear functionally and are irretrievable. ECMO survivors that come back after eight months and a year still have absent capillaries.

Dr. Bendixen: One of the alternatives to ECMO is, of course, long-term, high-pressure PEEP.

Dr. Peirce, what kind of problems do you see with this?

Dr. Peirce: Well, one has problems of instability of the circulatory system when one uses high levels of PEEP. One is likely to have instability of the circulatory system any time you go over 5-8 cm, and that means you need to monitor. If you are going to do a really good job, you will probably need to monitor such things as oxygen utilization in a patient, and not just cardiac output and things of that sort.

We have occasional patients who seem to respond very well to very high levels of PEEP, up to 40, and sometimes even 50 cm.

Patients who would not be candidates for ECMO, or for really anything else, seem to get by with this very high level, and you do seem to be able to manage them. I suspect that it does have a place.

Dr. Bendixen: What about it, Dr. Zapol?

Dr. Zapol: No, I think high levels of PEEP for short periods of time in carefully controlled situations, undoubtedly have a pretty useful place. We manage our controls that way, and I have not been impressed with a major difference in our controlled versus our ECMO survivors.

If you put it to the test on the same critically injured group of patients, my guess is, at present, we can show no significant difference.

Dr. Bendixen: We seem to get the impression that we are now talking about something that has become good technology.

What further technological developments are you looking towards, Dr. Hill?

Dr. Hill: Well, I did not say that it was good technology.

I mean, I would say that we are doing the best we can with the technology that we have. I think the technology I would like to see is a very small antithrombogenic, low-prime, high-efficiency membrane oxygenator, and it does not exist. It is a step toward the implantable lung. You can look at it either way you want. It would be a very good external or a primitive internal implanted lung.

When you get the technique down to the point where it is simple and safe, then the selection of the patient, and the idea of who should get it and should not, and the risk of the procedure, become much simpler to contend with.

What we have to contend with now is the balance of a series of patients treated with this system versus those treated with conventional therapy, of which the data on the latter is very very bad as some kind of a predictor.

If we were using something that was very simple and safe, then we would not have to worry about this.

I would like to discuss the question that was brought up before, the question of the fibrosis, etc, and how we alter the fibrosis. I have been unable, in my own mind, to sort out if it may be predetermined at almost the first or second day that a patient is drifting toward some pathological endpoint, regardless of what we do. It may be that all the patients reach a certain kind of pathology on day 1 or day 2, and then we start our intervention. It may be PEEP, it may be drugs, it may be oxygen, it may be something, but how much the current therapy interferes or changes the natural course of the disease, we don't know. It is not clear to me.

It may be that it has no effect at all. It may be that it is either helping us or hindering us, or it may be that it is predetermined at day 1 that this patient is going to end up with pulmonary fibrosis.

I see no easy way to get the answer, but one of the ways to have an alternative is to be able to put people on bypass extremely early, and very safely, to see if we can alter that course of the disease.

Dr. Bendixen: If we do all of these things, how many of the patients are awake and aware, and what are they feeling and what are they thinking about, Dr. Peirce?

Dr. Peirce: Well, the level of consciousness varies quite a bit, of course, but they can be quite fully awake. Patients may be able to communicate quite well with you during the time that they are on perfusion. They may express wishes of survival and communicate with you about feelings of discomfort and positions they would like to be in and so forth.

One is rather limited in communicating with the patients because they are intubated, and because they usually do require some sedation. I think the most alert patient is probably a patient like the one that one of our colleagues had, where the lung had reached near irreversible stages in about 17 days and this patient was actually sufficiently alert to take nourishment by the oral route. It was a question at that point of having to discontinue the perfusion. Therefore, one can have a very alert patient, but most of them are rather obtunded.

Dr. Zapol: We tend to paralyze cool, and give morphine to the patient, and at least the two survivors we can speak to are completely amnesic for about 45 or 50 days, and can remember nothing that went on during that time.

Dr. Bendixen: There must be enough survivors now so that we can begin to get some impression of exactly this.

Dr. Hill, what is your impression of that?

Dr. Hill: We have four survivors, and three of them remember nothing of what happened while they were really sick. The other one has the intimate details of it and this may be related to the mechanism by which he got into trouble.

He was in a knife fight and the last thing he remembered before he lost that fight was that there were two guys giving him a hard time, both with knives, and that he came to the San Francisco General Hospital where he had a laparotomy followed by a median sternotomy (the Market Street incision). He was opened completely. He had a cardiac arrest.

Ultimately, he recieved something like 120 bottles of blood at the San Francisco General Hospital before he came to us with ARI, and he had had half his liver removed. While on bypass, I entered his abdomen twice to try to control the bleeding from this liver area and ultimately we got him off bypass and he recovered. One of the things he kept saying was "You aren't going to kill me!" I think he thought he still was in the fight.

Anyway, he remembered a lot of little things that happened during perfusion and during the three to four weeks that he was really ill, but it has not had any long-term effects on his personality, he is back fighting again.

Dr. Bendixen: Realistically, what does it take in manpower to mount such an effort? Also, realistically, how quickly can you set up?

Dr. Hill: Well, once you are set up at the bedside, you need what I have; a nurse and a perfusion technician. Both these people are there all the time, and ordinarly we would always have a nurse there as well, so that, in manpower, we have one extra man.

In the beginning, there was myself, a nurse and Mr. Bramson. Now, in order to do the associated research that you must do during this procedure to know what we do right and what we do wrong, besides myself, there is another surgeon. I also have the support of two pulmonary physiologists, and have the support of two coagulationists. They don't have to be close by, but that depth is there if I want them. In essence, our patients are really managed by two or three physicians, and if I leave town or any of them leave town or half of them leave town, it does not mean that anything has to stop. It can go on.

All the nurses in our unit, which number 28, are familiar with how to take care of these patients and the technical problems associated with them. Also our five pump technicians are familiar with how to do everything. The house staff is probably the weakest link in this system, because they change and I have had some crazy things happen.

I mean, because the whole staff did not know, for example, that a pneumothorax in a person on ECMO is not as serious in a person with ARI, who you can lose in 2 minutes. On bypass you can have a pneumothorax, and you can take care of it at your leisure. If you ram a tube in the chest of these people, you will spend three days trying to stop them from bleeding.

So the weakest link in our system, I would say, is probably the house staff, only because they don't have the experience to look after these patients, but also because they cannot learn it in three to four months.

Dr. Bendixen: Well, what do our own local experts say? Janice, how quickly can you set up? Do you want to tell us that?

Ms. J. Follmer: About two hours.

Dr. Bendixen: Joanne, how many extra nurses do we need when we get one of these patients?

Ms. J. Lamb: About two.

Dr. Bendixen: Would you like to add to the list of what you might call the human patients' problems? What have we overlooked, if anything?

Audience Participant: I work with Dr. Zapol, so I can talk on his behalf.

I think that the essential ingredient is a hospital that will back you up with a blood bank, operating facilities, instantaneous operating equipment, a house staff that is not necessarily involved with fellows who are part of the team and continue to be part of the team. When you talk about one nurse, you are really talking about three nurses, and when you talk about one surgeon, you are talking about two surgeons, and when you talk about Dr. Zapol who masterminded the whole apparatus, he has two people who work with him who can replace him, if he is out of town or at least be in contact with him.

It requires a tremendous effort and backup—hematology, infectious disease pathology, and the kind of things that most hospitals have routinely. Also people who are specialized in pulmonary pathology and are interested in what Dr. Hill discussed, which are the research aspects of it, so you can do immunofibrinogens or a pulmonary physiology group that will help you not only with ventilation abnormalities, but perhaps discuss with you distribution of flow, distributions of gas, bronchoscopic capabilities. I think that ECMO is a perhaps a larger game than even Dr. Hill made it sound like.

Maybe we make a meal of it up in Boston; I don't know.

Dr. Bendixen: Dr. Peirce?

Dr. Peirce: I think this is a very good question. I have been appalled at how long it takes to get one of these things started, particularly with the National Protocol Data to fulfil. Because of this we have set up an emergency perfusion apparatus, which is pneumatically driven and on a cart that we can take anywhere in the hospital, and all of the things that are required for cannulating and perfusing are on the cart. With this cart, one can realistically, having made the decision, be ready to perfuse as soon as the surgeon has the cannulae in place, and that is probably realistically about 30 minutes. So that it can be initiated in quite a short time, but in order to do this, you have to think out every single item that is required, and it has to be readily available for instant operation. This, of course, presumes that you are going to start your perfusion without using whole blood.

Now, as far as the personnel are concerned, there are never enough. I think that is the answer to the question.

There have never been enough. To start out with, it takes something more than one nurse there all the time, and that means that you have to do it practically in a mileu, where you have a fairly large body of nurses, who are trained to help out periodically, where you have to do things with the patient. If you try to do it in an isolated area, you are licked. It is just almost impossible.

Then you need two nurses *all* the time. You need a technician and need the doctor, or a well-trained pump technician there all the time with the present set-up, plus all of the other people who have been talked about, like engineers and physiologists and so forth, that are essential. But you cannot really count them in as whole people all the time.

Dr. Bendixen: A final brief comment.

Dr. Zapol: I can answer your question regarding how long it takes.

We pulled the data on all the National Heart and Lung Institute's ECMO patients on the first two years and looked at the time between randomization and ECMO, and Dr. Hill has the fastest time–4 hours (mean) and it runs to about 8 hours in the newer groups.

So it is about 8 hours from knowing you have to absolutely perfuse the patient, in a group that knows about it, and in a set-up that does this kind of thing for a living. So if you are not in the business, it will take you two or three times the regular length of time, which is a big problem.

Dr. Bendixen: I think we will let Dr. Zapol's statement be the last word.

Dr. Bregman: Thank you, Dr. Bendixen. I have one closing remark. I would like to thank all of our distinguished panelists for their contributions and I would particularly like to thank Dr. Reemtsma and Dr. Bendixen for their excellent moderating jobs.

Index

(Page numbers in **boldface type** indicate tables and illustrations.)